Great progress has been made in heart imaging techniques in recent years. Cardiologists can see the heart in minute detail.

 80

*If treatment is started one hour after the pain starts, the extent of damage to the heart might only be in the region of 5% and the death rate greatly reduced.* ▶ 78

*Cardiac massage is carried out by placing the heel of both palms on the sternum and applying pressure* **80** *to* **100** *times a minute.*

 67

**Smoking** *increases the risk of heart attack or angina pectoris* ▶ 100 *by 70%.*

*The heart weighs*
*8 to 10 ounces;*
*it beats 50 to 100*
*times a minute,*
*100,000 times a day*
*for 80 years or more...*

 54

# Trials have shown that small doses of aspirin taken over a long period reduc the risk of coronary thrombosis by between 23 and 44%.

 78

High blood pressure, smoking and alcohol, high cholesterol levels, diabetes, stress, obesity, sedentary lifestyle – if combined, these risk factors are even more likely to predispose people to heart disease. Today they are better understood and can be monitored.

 108

blood pressure

# How your
exertion        pacemaker   cardiology
# heart works
scanner        thrombolytics
fibrillation

Véronique Warnod
Carole Émile

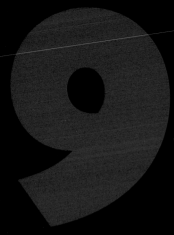**9** pints of blood are pumped by the heart every minute. ▶ 56

A *sudden* *sensation of tightness* **in the chest, spreading into the arm, a feeling of** *anxiety,* *cold sweats* **... symptoms that warn of the ▶ 66 onset of a heart attack. It is fatal in 30 % of cases.**

**60,000** miles of arteries and veins are irrigated by our blood. ▶ 59

# 'As mine on hers, so hers is set on mine'

*Romeo and Juliet*
**Shakespeare**

 21

# 50 . 100 to
## beats a minute – a normal heart rate.

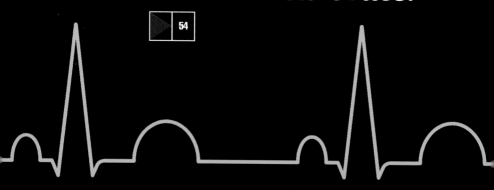

| 54 |

## Look after your heart

Vary your diet, don't use too much salt. Roughly one person in 500 is predisposed to clogging of the coronary arteries caused by too high a level of fat in the blood. Blood tests help to detect high cholesterol levels.

 | 112 |

## War in the arteries

A small balloon is inflated to crush the fatty deposits obstructing the artery. The killer blockage is removed. A metal net is put in position to help avoid a recurrence of the obstruction ... Heart specialists now have an increasingly effective range of methods for carrying out angioplasty.

 | 82 |

*Today, all branches of science are working together to save our hearts: chemistry, biology, physics, genetics ...*

 90

**The first heart transplant took place over 30 years ago.**

The technique is well perfected now but donors are in short supply.

 88

## Defibrillator implants

Automatic defibrillators can now be fully implanted. However, this is new technology and extremely expensive. Consequently, while they are likely to benefit patients in the long term they have not yet been widely introduced into hospitals.

 87

## Stress

Whether physical or emotional, stress increases the heart's workload.

 108

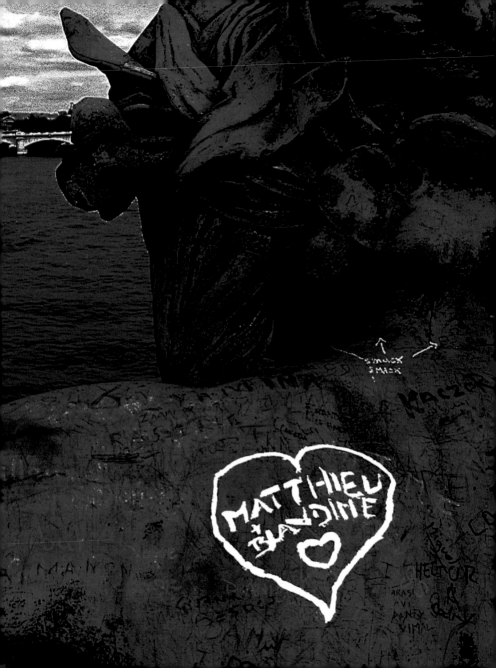

'The heart that has truly loved never forgets.'

Thomas Moore

# Cardiac arrest is the cause of more than 140,000 deaths every year in the UK, 400,000 in Europe, 500,000 in the United States.

Across the world, cardiac arrest affects men more than women, although it is still the biggest killer of women.

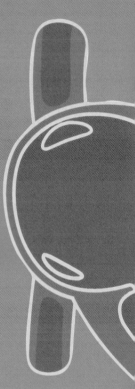

A grafted artery straddles the obstruction and establishes a bypass that restores circulation: heart bypass operations are very straightforward today.

*Coronary thrombosis, heart rate disorders – every minute that passes means* **10%** *less chance of survival. After* **4 minutes** *without resuscitation, the brain is starved of blood and may suffer irreversible damage.*  67

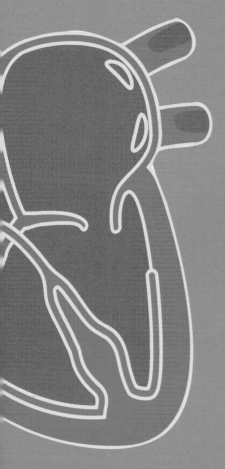

## Survival tips to help gain a few vital minutes.

**1.** Call for help by dialling 999.
**2.** If unconscious, shout loudly, or tap the patient's cheek.
**3.** Check the airway is clear.
**4.** Start mouth-to-mouth resuscitation and cardiac massage.
**5.** If conscious, give the patient an aspirin to chew.

67

The semi-automatic **defibrillator** increases survival chances by **20%** to **50%**. With a little bit of training, anyone is capable of using it. Press a button and an **electric shock** sets the heart back into its normal rhythm. The cost: **£1,500**, the price of a life.  ▶ 87

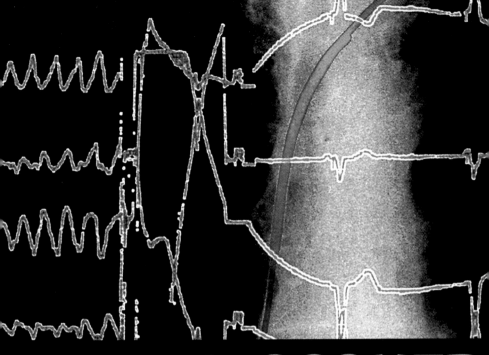

# DISCOVER

AT THE CENTRE OF THE HUMAN BODY IS THE HEART,
HOME OF THE EMOTIONS, THE SOUL AND A SYMBOL OF LOVE.
DOCTORS HAVE STUDIED THE HEART FOR CENTURIES, BUT IT WAS NOT UNTIL
THE 20TH CENTURY THAT SURGEONS ATTEMPTED TO OPERATE ON THE HEART.
SINCE THEN OUR KNOWLEDGE OF HOW THE HEART WORKS
HAS GROWN AT AN ASTONISHING PACE.

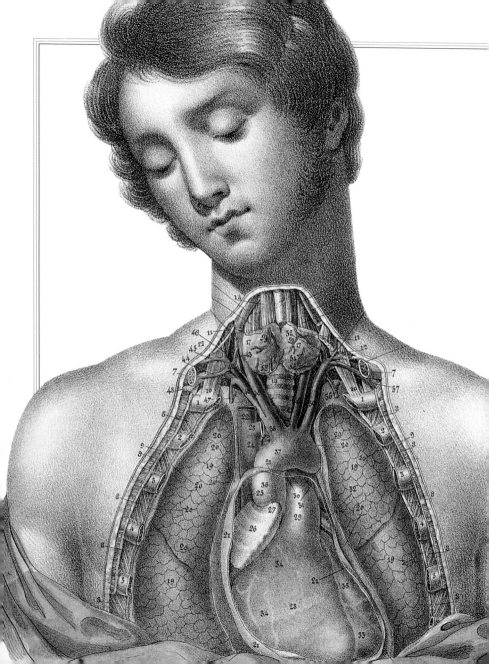

**P**hysically, the heart is just another organ, a muscle, but a vital one as it maintains life. With every beat, it sends oxygen-rich blood to the billions of cells that form the body. Study the prehistoric paintings in caves spread around Europe and you will see that hunters in the Palaeolithic age made the heart their target when in pursuit of game; the paintings depict arrows converging with deadly intent upon the chests of their prey. The heart, as the centre of all living animals, has been endowed with a sacred symbolism and revered for its life-giving properties from the very earliest civilisations.

## THE HEART AS A GIVER OF LIFE

The heart was fundamental to the concept of human life and death for many ancient civilisations. According to the beliefs of the Ancient Egyptians, when a person died, they were summoned to appear before the gods in order to prove that they had led a good life. Their heart was weighed on scales. If it proved to be as light as a feather and so without sin, then Thot, the scribe of the gods, wrote out a sentence of acquittal and Horus took them by the hand and led them away to the after-life alongside his father Osiris.

**OPEN HEART**

*Early 19th century representation of the organs in the chest as they were understood at the time (Manual of Anatomy, 1825).*

Thus, at the court of the dead, innocence or guilt was determined by the weight of the heart. It was removed from the body by the embalmers, and put in a jar. Its place was taken inside the mummy by a sacred insect that took the form of a beetle made of stone. By replacing a heart burdened with sin, the beetle was supposed to confer certain advantages on the deceased, protecting them from cold and hunger. The Egyptians removed the heart from the body in order to place it under the protection of the gods. They believed that it was the cause of all the difficulties that people experienced in their lives.

## THE HEART AS A VESSEL FOR KNOWLEDGE

In Ancient Egypt, the heart was also regarded as the seat of learning, or intelligence. The Egyptians worshipped knowledge, believing that it made cultured and educated men superior to the rest of the population. Men such as the scribe who had spent long hours studying could be employed in any form of state administration, thus avoiding the physical labour carried out by ordinary workers. Instead, from his elevated intellectual vantage point replete with knowledge, the scholar could supervise the work of other men. However, knowledge and wisdom were not enough to keep health problems at bay!

Egyptian medicine went hand in hand with religion and its representatives, the priests. To cure their patients, doctors often resorted to magic formulas, and incantations were thought

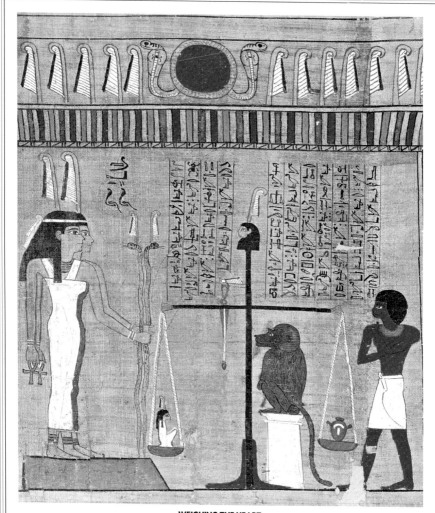

**WEIGHING THE HEART**

*During judgement, or psychostasis, whereby it was decided whether the deceased might enter the kingdom of Osiris, it was the heart that gave evidence of the deceased person's good and bad actions. The lighter the heart, the better the chances (Book of the Dead, an Egyptian papyrus).*

to enhance the power of their remedies. The patient would help, if able, by reciting: 'Come, remedy, come, you who chase away sickness from my heart and limbs ...' In this way magic made up for the lack of anatomical knowledge surprising in a people who practised dissection of bodies.

The extent of the Ancient Egyptians' medical knowledge was mainly restricted to the network of veins and channels that they discovered in the course of their dissections. They believed that the large veins and arteries going to the various parts of the body all began from the heart: 'It contains vessels for every limb; wherever the doctor places his fingers, on the head, back of the head, hands, arms or legs, he comes across the heart, because its vessels lead to all parts of the body. That is how its voice spreads to all parts of the body.'

Through this interpretation of the vascular system, the Egyptians attributed explanations for the causes of many ailments that had completely different origins, for example rheumatism: 'The vessels clog up, become hot, harden and are subject to itching; they have to be strengthened and soothed with ointments and poultices.' A pale face, constipation, distended stomach – according to the Egyptians, everything stemmed from the heart. They concocted remedies for relieving these troubles from the plants and animals that they had around them. Despite their omnipotence, even the gods did not escape the problems of illness suffered by mere mortals. The Egyptians believed that the gods were beset by the same kinds of ailments as those experienced by humans.

## THE OLD TESTAMENT: CONVERTING HEARTS OF STONE INTO HEARTS OF FLESH

The concept of the heart of stone, used to describe someone who is insensitive to the misfortunes of others or incapable of expressing benevolent feelings, appears in the Old Testament. The prophet Ezekiel announces that God is going to place his love in even the hardest of men's hearts through 'spiritual transplantation'; God states: 'I shall give you a new heart and shall place in you a new spirit; I shall remove the heart of stone from your flesh. I shall place my Spirit within you.' The prophet Jeremiah adds that it is not enough to say: 'This is the temple of the Eternal.' Above all, the bible teaches that we must not spill the blood of the innocent, we must be charitable to the bereaved and to strangers, for the real temple of the Lord is the heart of a pious man. God is present wherever a loving gesture takes place and especially in the hearts of men.

On the subject of the need to fill a heart with a sentiment of some kind, presumably goodness, Martin Luther, the German religious reformer said, 'The human heart is like a millstone in a mill: when you put wheat under it, it turns and grinds and bruises the wheat to flour; if you put no wheat, it still grinds on, but then 'tis itself it grinds and wears away.'

## THE SACRIFICIAL HEART

In 1519, the Conquistadors discovered Mexico, the Aztec capital that ruled a powerful empire. The European soldiers saw only a cruel, bloodthirsty people, who sacrificed prisoners on pyramid altars by tearing out their hearts with sharp-edged stones. The origin of these rites was very ancient. They were carried out in honour of the gods, particularly the Sun god, who, to the Aztecs, was the source of life on Earth.

The last of a wave of migrants from the north of the continent, the Aztecs spent centuries wandering in search of their promised land. As they made their way south, travelling through many different kingdoms, they tried to form alliances with the peoples along the way but were driven away each time. Continuing their search for a homeland, they finally arrived in the heart of an area of marshland at dawn one day. According to legend, the priests who were guiding them experienced a revelation when they arrived there. The holy men reported seeing a stone turn into a prickly pear with an eagle astride it, its head pointing towards the place where they should settle. This sign from heaven was interpreted as confirmation that they could legitimately occupy the territory, which they named Tenochtitlan, 'the place of the stone prickly pear', so they forced the inhabitants to flee, and built a city. The story of the stone echoes that of another tale, centred upon a previous battle. The Aztecs had attacked a number of neighbouring cities and during one of these raids, a rival chief had been captured, his heart sacrificed and his body thrown into the lagoon. The heart had turned to stone and a prickly pear began to grow, prophetically marking the site of the future Tenochtitlan. This explains why, in Aztec writing symbols, the fruit of the prickly pear represents the hearts of victims sacrificed to the Sun.

### AZTEC SACRIFICES

*The Aztecs carried out human sacrifices to return strength to the sun after its nocturnal journeying, and thus delay the end of the world. The hearts of sacrificial victims were torn out and burned while the blood, the precious vital liquid, flowed down the steps of the sanctuary-pyramid (16th century).*

The city's founding myth was therefore based on a sacrificial ideology, and human sacrifice became vital to the survival of the Aztec people. But all this was to change after the Spanish conquest.

For the Aztecs the sacrificing of human hearts was simply paying the tribute of human lives demanded by the all-powerful Sun. Through their warlike vision, they viewed the world as a place to be conquered and dominated. Human sacrifice was used to maintain their very ancient tribal heritage. However, the invaders, the strongly Catholic Spanish, were disgusted by the rites and set about trying to change the blood thirsty way of life of the people of Tenochtitlan.

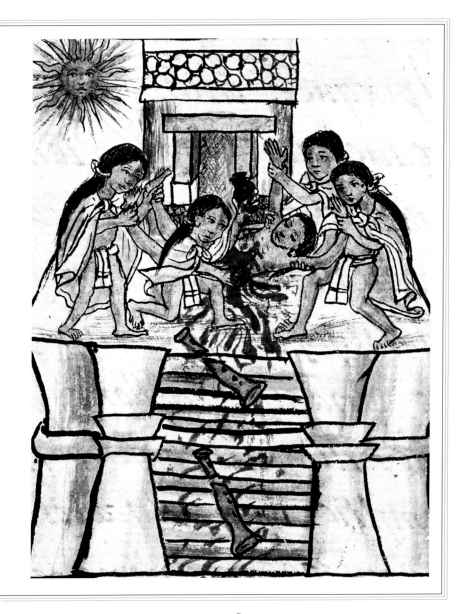

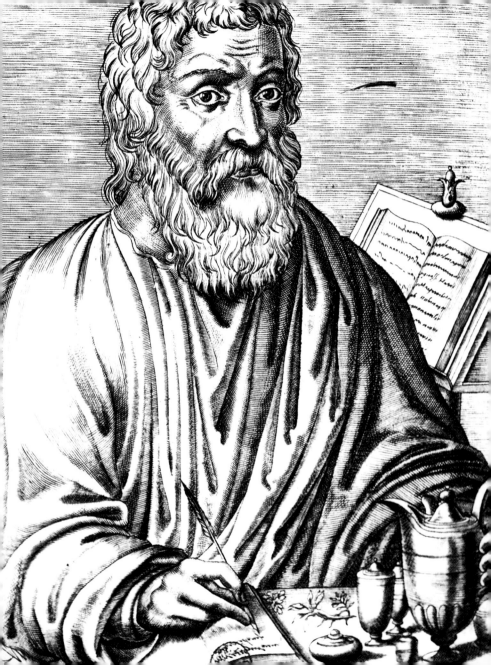

## THE HEART RULES

As centuries passed, people attributed emotive functions to the heart. It became the sea of feelings and of love. In Shakespeare's *Romeo and Juliet*, Romeo talks of the bonds of the heart that unite him with Juliet: 'As mine on hers, so hers is set on mine.' Today, the symbolic forces surrounding the heart are just as strong. Linked with blood-stirring terms such as courage, morality and a sense of honour and duty, the importance of the heart is clear.

With these values being attributed to the heart, it is not surprising that we have a predilection for heart-shaped pendants, brooches and other jewels. For some, they act as lucky charms, for others they ward off the evil eye, bring luck in love or protect against illness.

The Egyptians of 4,000 years ago already had an inkling of the role of the heart when they compared the aorta to the great river Nile that irrigates their country, and when they likened a heart attack to the heart in the act of 'forgetting'. The Chinese formulated a similar view of blood circulation. Unfortunately, Eastern medicine had very little influence on its Western counterpart because of linguistic differences, geographical distance and differing beliefs and philosophies, which were often widely opposed to those of the West. For a long time European doctors believed that arteries carried air because they were found to be empty after death.

## THE FIRST STEPS OF WESTERN MEDICINE

Hippocrates (*c.*460 BC – *c.*377 BC), the Greek physician, was the first to describe the heart as a muscle and to comment on the body's humours, especially the blood. The humours were the four bodily fluids believed to contribute towards a person's temperament: blood, bile, melancholy and phlegm. Hippocrates also made a thorough and systematic study of the symptoms of certain diseases. He gave an excellent description of the symptoms of acute cardiac insufficiency and pulmonary oedema, for which he formulated a 'treatment for water on the lungs', based on bloodletting or phlebotomy, which saved many lives. Diuretics, which form part of current treatment for cardiac insufficiency, work according to the same principle: they ease the heart's workload by reducing the volume of fluid in the circulation.

**HIPPOCRATES**

*His moral code concerning the art of medicine has been passed to posterity. Today, throughout the world, every day and in all languages, young doctors still take the Hippocratic oath.*

Hippocrates' treatments, involving these sometimes spectacularly life-saving bloodlettings, were only abandoned in the 19th century.

Borrowing from Hippocrates' theories, the work of the Greek physician Galen (*c.*131 – *c.*201) was also based on the existence of four humours, four basic qualities (heat, cold, wetness and dryness) and three spirits located in the liver, heart and brain. Although today we know that this theory has no scientific value, it was adopted by the Arabs and was prevalent throughout the Middle Ages, strongly influencing medical thinking until the 17th century. Galen studied anatomy by dissecting animals and was the first to refute the idea that blood crossed from the right side of the heart to the left via a leaky membrane.

## THE REAL BEGINNINGS OF ANATOMY

As a result of Hippocrates' teachings, the heart was considered to be the inviolable seat of the soul, so any attempt to physically tamper with it was taboo, and heart surgery was forbidden. It was only as an indirect result of the Renaissance and the tremendous artistic movement that accompanied it that medicine finally moved forward. The artists of the period realised how important it was to have a sound knowledge of anatomy in order to reproduce the wonders of the human body in sculpture and painting.

Leonardo da Vinci (1452–1519) was perhaps the first to embark on a serious anatomical and functional study of the heart. In his sketchbooks, he depicted the heart and its valve system very accurately, and later applied the same principle to a design for hydraulic pump valves. He made his observations during trips to Florence and Rome between 1503 and 1516, where he was able to carry out dissections on corpses in hospitals, a practice that had only recently become accepted. Andre Vesale (1514–1564), a Flemish teacher of dissection, used the procedure to explain in detail the general structure of the heart and the anatomy of the veins and coronary arteries. Gradually, the dissection of corpses became legally acceptable. The Italian anatomist Giambattista Morgagni (1682–1771) developed the science of clinical anatomy, which enabled doctors to link the symptoms of illness they saw when they examined a patient with the known anatomical appearance of abnormalities within the body. In this way Morgagni described the hardening and shrinking of the coronary arteries, which we now know as atherosclerosis. Later, in 1772, William Heberden (1710–1801) gave members of the London School of Medicine a presentation of angina pectoris, named from the Latin *angina* (to strangle) and *pectoris* (chest).

**THE ANATOMY OF THE HEART**

*One of the first anatomical representations of the heart and its blood vessels, drawn by Leonardo da Vinci, who made more than 800 drawings of the human body.*

## THE DISCOVERY OF BLOOD CIRCULATION

It was William Harvey (1578–1657), physician to King James I and fellow of the Royal College of Physicians, who discovered the circulation of the blood. He found that oxygen-rich arterial blood is pumped by the left ventricle of the heart into the aorta, which distributes it to arteries throughout the body. After supplying all the tissues of the body, the blood, now carrying carbon

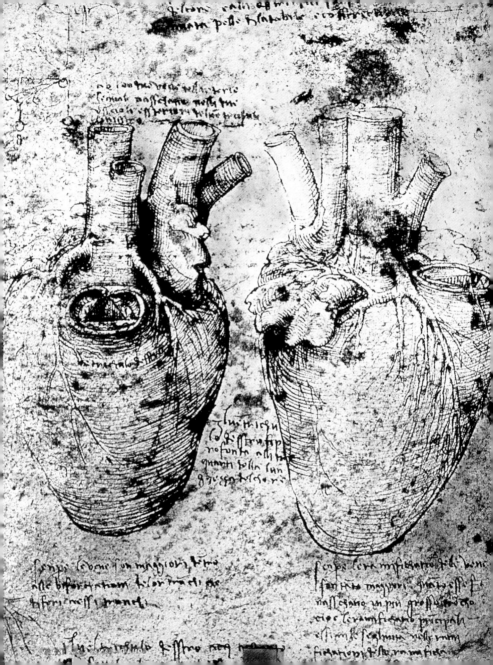

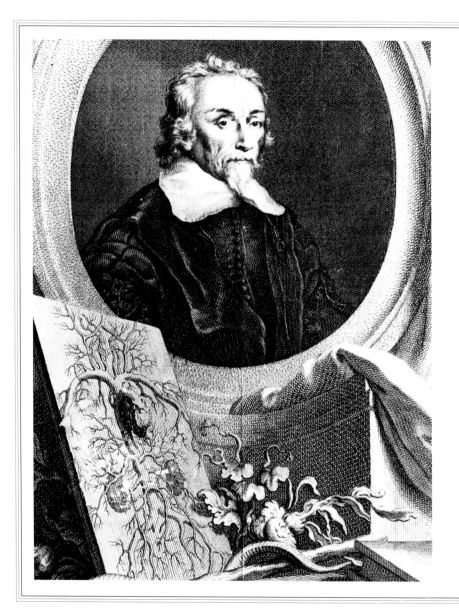

dioxide (the 'waste product' created when the body's tissues have used the oxygen), is then returned through the veins to the right atrium of the heart, then the right ventricle, which sends it to the lungs to exchange the carbon dioxide for oxygen. Returning from the lungs through the pulmonary veins, the blood reaches the left atrium before returning to the left ventricle, from where it started its journey. The Italian doctor and anatomist Marcello Malpighi (1628–1694) confirmed Harvey's discoveries by studying blood circulation in frogs. He also discovered that our lungs are full of microscopic blood vessels thin enough for oxygen to be absorbed by the blood cells in them.

**WILLIAM HARVEY**

*Harvey is considered to be the father of modern cardiology. His discovery of the circulation of the blood eclipsed all previous knowledge of the heart.*

Harvey managed to complete a full diagram of blood circulation , and of the lungs, thanks to the invention of the microscope, which enabled him to observe the capillaries, the tiniest vessels which supply blood to every part of the body. However, his theory was not well received by university doctors, who continued to recommend bloodletting according to the precepts of Galenic medicine. After all, how could Galen have been wrong? A quarrel broke out between those who believed in Harvey's theory of circulation and those who did not ...

## AIDS TO DIAGNOSIS

In 1625, following Harvey's discovery of circulation, a renowned Venetian doctor, Santorio Santorio (1561–1636), whose name is often seen in the Latin form Sanctorius, invented the pulse timer, which enabled doctors to calculate heart rate. However, the next two hundred years saw very little progress in the physical examination of patients until René Laennec (1781–1826) published an article in which he described the various stages of examination: inspection, auscultation (listening), palpation and percussion. For most of the medical establishment, this systematic form of examination reduced the doctor's art to simple mechanics. Despite this, René Laennec continued his search for better methods of hearing the heartbeat. One day, he rolled up a sheet of paper and placed it between his ear and his patient's chest. For the first time, he could clearly hear the heart and sounds of breathing. He improved on his idea and, in 1819, presented his design to the Paris School of Medicine. He had just designed and invented the first stethoscope. This indispensable instrument is still used daily by all doctors, its design having changed little in two hundred years. After the successful invention of the stethoscope many other methods of examining the heart were developed.

In 1869, Étienne Jules Marey (1830–1904) invented the sphygmograph, a device which could measure the pulse and register heart rate. In Vienna, in 1881, Victor Basch (1863–1944) designed a sphygmomanometer, consisting of an elastic pocket attached to a manometer, which he used to measure blood pressure. Then, in 1896, the Italian, Scipione Riva-Rocci, equipped the sphygmomanometer with an inflatable armband, so pioneering the modern method of measuring blood pressure. However, the prognostic significance of blood pressure was not to be fully understood for several decades to come, and the first drugs to combat high blood pressure were not developed until after the Second World War.

In 1895, a German physicist, Wilhelm Röntgen (1845–1923), discovered X-rays and their direct application, radiography. The first X-ray he took was of his wife's hand. A year later, another physicist, the Frenchman Henri Becquerel (1852–1908), discovered nuclear radioactivity. 1934 saw a great leap forward with the production of artificial radioactivity by Frédéric Joliot and Irène Joliot-Curie. This was the first step towards heart scintigraphy, a diagnostic technique that uses radiation to produce a picture of an internal body organ. In 1906, using a machine he had invented himself, a Dutch physiologist, Willem Einthoven (1860–1927), managed to record the heart's electrical activity; in other words, he invented the first electrocardiogram or ECG. He received the Nobel Prize in 1924 for this remarkable achievement. One discovery followed another, but there was one area of medicine that remained isolated from progress until almost half way through the 18th century, surgery.

## FROM BARBER TO SURGEON

Following a decision by the Council of Latran in 1215, monks who practised medicine in the Middle Ages were forced to give up their role as surgeons, as the Church forbade them from attending to the sick if there were women present. Barbers, who were used to wielding razors and scissors, took over from the monks and became barber-surgeons, but they did not have the knowledge or training of the monks, who studied Greek and Latin manuscripts or works translated from Arabic. Some university-qualified doctors tried to rectify this deficiency by creating Schools of Surgery attached to hospitals, but they were keen to retain their privileges and so restricted the training, prohibiting barbers from following university medical courses. As a result, very few barber-surgeons managed to forge any sort of reputation.

There was, however, one exception, a certain Ambroise Paré (1509–1590). In 1563, having become a Court Surgeon, he published the enormous work that was the first book of medicine to be printed in French. In France and abroad, his *Oeuvres*, a huge number of treatises, rapidly became a reference book for surgeons. All aspects of diagnosis and treatment of diseases requiring surgery were covered, in particular the procedure for tying off arteries (ligaturing), a process which Ambroise Paré invented. With the help of this huge practical manual, barber-surgeons were now able to emerge from their subordinate position. This took longer in the UK than on the

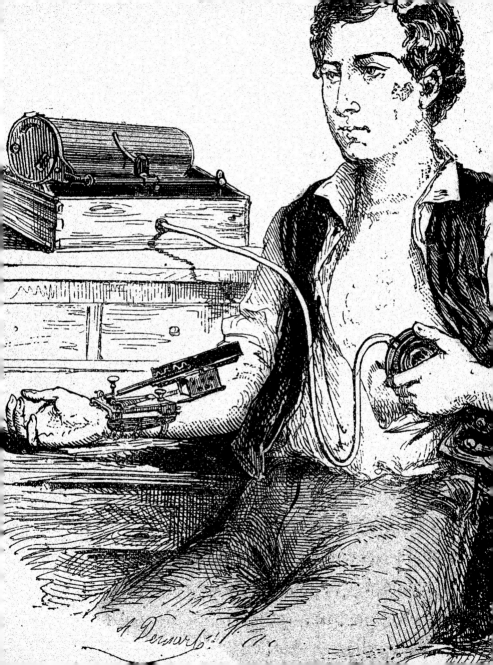

continent, and while the Company of Surgeons was founded in 1745 it was not granted a Royal Charter, raising surgeons to the same status as doctors, until 1840.

## THE HEART IS NO LONGER SACRED

During the 19th century, wounds to the heart were not operated on. A great German surgeon of the time, Theodore Billroth (1829–1894), stated: 'Any surgeon who attempts to suture a heart wound can expect to lose the respect of his colleagues for ever.' However, in 1896, in Frankfurt-am-Main, Professor Rehn decided to operate on a dying patient who had been wounded in the heart the day before, and whose blood circulation was weakening rapidly. When he opened the pericardium (the membrane surrounding the heart), a jet of blood escaped from the space between it and the heart wall itself. Using sterilised cloths and his finger to stem the loss of blood, Professor Rehn managed to stop the haemorrhage from a hole in the left ventricle. The heart did not stop beating and the wounded patient was still alive. Rehn placed two stitches in the heart muscle and the heart took up its regular beat. A month later, the patient had recovered and left hospital. News of this operation spread rapidly through the surgical world. The aura of mystery and inviolability surrounding the heart had finally been removed and at last the way was open to heart surgery.

## EARLY SUCCESSES IN HEART SURGERY

Heart surgery is a recent phenomenon , but its progress has been dazzling. Following a few faltering steps at the start of the 20th century, it really exploded into life in the early 1970s.

It started in Boston, in 1938, when the first blood vessel ligatures were carried out, using silk thread on an arterial duct. But real thoracic surgery did not take place until after the Second World War, and by this time it had the advantage of three fundamental discoveries: anaesthesia, via the installation of a tube in the trachea (windpipe) to provide artificial respiration while a patient was unconscious; blood transfusion; and the use of antibiotics (penicillin) to combat infections after surgery. These three major improvements meant that blood vessels entering or leaving the heart could be repaired with a simple suture.

In 1948, doctors became more daring and, for the first time, cut into the heart to dilate a shrunken valve. The first open heart operations did not take place for another ten years. Such operations require the body to tolerate a non-beating heart for much longer than the normal three minutes. The patient therefore had to be placed temporarily in non-physiological conditions. Two procedures were used to achieve this: cooling the body to 28°C and hyperbaric oxygenation, which involves increasing the concentration of oxygen in the blood. These techniques have now been superseded, but there was nevertheless some spin-off, as hypothermia is still a key element in heart bypass operations.

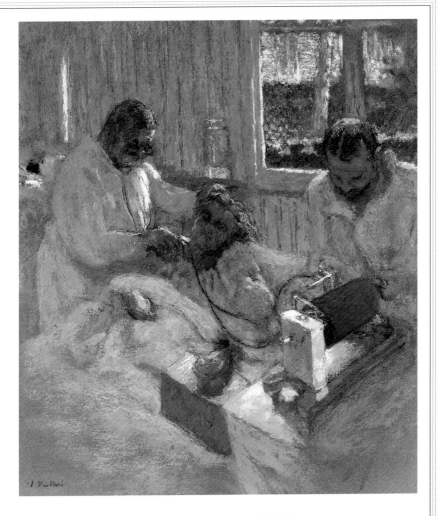

**THE CARDIOLOGIST AND HIS ASSISTANT**

*At the start of the 20th century, there was such progress in cardiology that doctors were finally able to cure certain heart pathologies. They were helped by increasingly effective instruments (Vuillard, c.1917).*

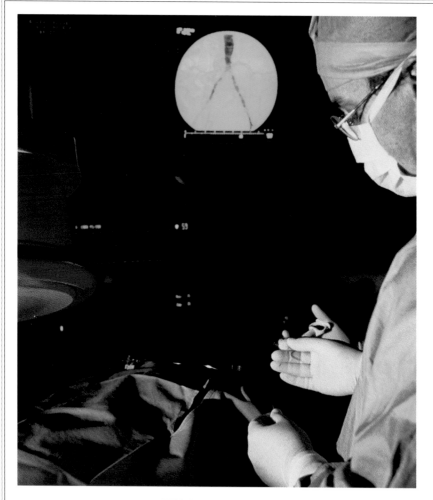

**THE CARDIOLOGIST AT WORK**

*Nowadays, medical imaging enables surgeons to carry out operations*
*with great accuracy. Probes are used to project pictures of*
*diseased arteries on to a screen*
*(angiography of the aorta and femoral arteries).*

## PROBLEMS ARE OVERCOME

Initially, heart surgery was concerned with repairing heart malformations. One important step has been the development of valve surgery. The idea of replacing damaged valves with human valves taken from corpses developed in the early 1960's, but there were obvious difficulties involved with setting up a valve bank supplied by human tissue. Surgeons therefore had to use animal valves, taken from pigs, or metal valves. Such surgery had its limitations. After eight or ten years, calcification or degeneration occurred almost inevitably, requiring further surgery to replace valve prostheses. Another major problem, heart failure, was almost completely eradicated in less than a quarter of a century with the invention of a device that artificially compensated for a weak heart rate: the heart stimulator, or pacemaker. The first pacemaker was fitted to a 76 year old man in 1958. At that time, the device weighed several dozen kilograms and sat on a trolley. Nowadays, a pacemaker weighs only a few grams and is implanted inside the body in a routine operation.

## THE HEART BYPASS OPERATION: A GIANT LEAP FORWARD

Surgery made enormous progress in the treatment of angina pectoris and coronary thrombosis (which can lead to a heart attack), using coronary artery bypass and angioplasty techniques. A narrowed or blocked coronary artery that can no longer provide sufficient blood, and so oxygen, to the heart muscle, can be bypassed. A length of the patient's leg vein (saphenous vein) is removed and then sewn to the aorta and to a point below the blockage or stenosis (narrowing). Blood flow then bypasses the diseased part of the artery. The first bypass operation was carried out in 1964 by Edward Garrett in Cleveland, United States, using a leg vein for the graft. Today, several thousand bypass operations are carried out in the UK each year.

Another type of operation, coronary artery angioplasty, is helping to improve prospects for patients who have suffered a coronary thrombosis. The first operation of this type was carried out in Switzerland in 1977 by Andreas Gruntzig. Angioplasty consists of dilating the coronary arteries using a small balloon, and is today considered to be the quickest form of treatment for a heart attack. It has certainly reaped the benefits of recent technological and pharmacological progress. The risk of the artery becoming blocked again after the balloon angioplasty is reduced by the placing of a stent, a type of splint designed to keep the vessel fully open. In addition, an accompanying prescription of new and highly effective platelet anti-aggregation drugs, such as abciximab, improves the outcome of the technique even further, reducing the threat of recurring obstruction by 15 per cent.

## HEART TRANSPLANTS

Professor Christiaan Barnard was a pioneering heart surgeon who decided to attempt the impossible: transplant the beating heart from a brain-dead patient. In December 1967, in Cape Town, South Africa, he successfully carried out the first heart transplant in the history of medicine. The transplant patient, a 54-year-old man, survived for 18 days after the operation.

From then on, further attempts were made, but all ended in failure due to rejection of the transplanted heart. There was one exception in France: the Frenchman Emmanuel Vitria lived for 20 years with a transplanted heart. It was not until 1983, with the introduction of cyclosporin, a highly effective immunosuppressant, that the success rate improved significantly. But the lack of donors has prompted researchers to look more closely at xenografting – the grafting of organs from other species.

**AN IMPLANTED DEFIBRILLATOR**

*The heart of a patient suffering from ventricular fibrillation is given an electric shock by this tiny device, which enables it to return to its normal rhythm. Without this, such rhythm disorders can be fatal.*

The earliest research into mechanical hearts began in 1931 and was the result of collaboration between Nobel prize-winner Alexis Carrel and the aviator Charles Lindbergh, who had become very wealthy. In 1957, researchers kept a dog alive for two hours with a mechanical heart. Fourteen years later, a calf fitted with a mechanical heart survived for three months. Since 1985, animals fitted with a mechanical heart have survived for at least a year. In 1969, two attempts to fit mechanical hearts to humans ended in failure, with both patients surviving only a few hours after the operation. Research continues, and more and more sophisticated mechanical hearts are being produced. Two lines of research are favoured: temporary ventricular support, which is already in use to help patients get through a difficult stage; and the full, definitive, permanently fitted artificial heart, which has still not been perfected.

## DRUGS TO SUPPORT THE HEART

Over the last thirty years, the wonders of heart surgery have provoked both amazement and hope, but such achievements could not have occurred without the support of pharmacology. Drugs such as beta-blockers and calcium channel blockers enable the weary heart to work just as efficiently with less effort. In the 1990s, statins opened up new ways of preventing cardiovascular disease. These new molecules, by lowering cholesterol in the blood, can help prevent the appearance of atherosclerosis or restrict its development, thereby reducing the likelihood of heart attacks and strokes.

Research carried out in Framingham, in the United States, in the late 1940s showed the main risk factors involved in the development of heart disease. These are high blood pressure,

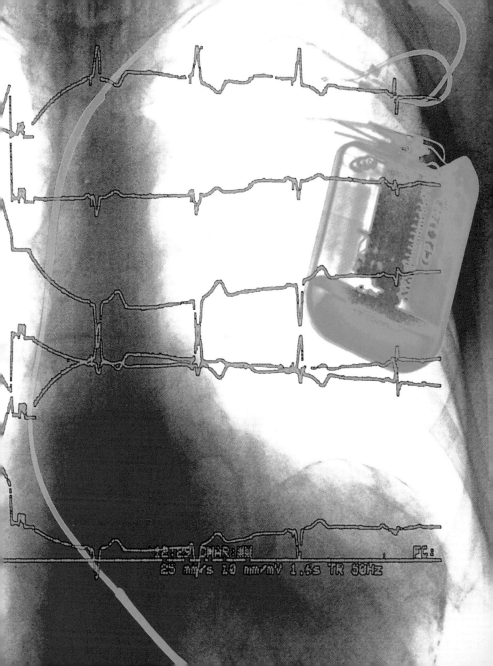

smoking, high cholesterol in the blood, diabetes, being of the male sex, old age and family history of early vascular disease. Since then, the medical profession has tried to develop medicinal and non-medicinal strategies for dealing with these risk factors. From large-scale use of drugs to lower blood pressure to wide-ranging research showing the benefits of cholesterol-lowering drugs in heart patients and healthy individuals, the epic story of treatments to fight atherosclerosis goes on and on. The benefits of using statins in primary and secondary prevention treatments have been well proven in the last few years.

## THE DISCOVERY OF ASPIRIN

Commonly used for many purposes today, aspirin is also effective in helping prevent heart disease. It was discovered a century ago, but its beneficial effects on the heart have only been known for thirty years. The abilities of willow bark to relieve pain and fever have been known for centuries: the leaves of *Salix alba* figured in the Sumerian pharmacopoeia, and in the Middle Ages, the leaves of meadowsweet (*Spiraea ulmaria*) were used to relieve the same symptoms. Scholars, pharmacists and chemists studied these plants over the years, until a young chemist working in the Bayer laboratories perfected the drug that was to become one of the most commonly used in the world. On 1 February 1899, Bayer launched a new product onto the market called Aspirin. Another seventy years went by before Sir John Vane discovered that aspirin also reduces the formation of blood clots. By paralysing blood platelets, it prevents them from sticking together, which is the first stage of coagulation. Very small doses, much smaller than those needed for pain relief, are enough to protect the blood vessels. When administered over a long period, aspirin helps to prevent coronary thromboses and strokes.

## CARDIOLOGY: FROM ONE INNOVATION TO ANOTHER

Medicine has seen more changes in the last forty years than in the previous thirty centuries: progress in anaesthesia, the gene revolution, the discovery of blood and tissue groups making blood transfusion and organ transplants possible ... the list goes on! And the revolution that we are seeing in cardiology embraces every branch of science: radiology, with progress in angiography and MRA (magnetic resonance angiography), the most recent offshoot of MRI (magnetic resonance imaging); surgery, with minimally-invasive surgery and 'plastic surgery' for coronary arteries; chemistry, with drug development leading to the treatment and prevention of atherosclerosis; physics, with the use of the laser; genetics, which has led to transplanting and new blood vessel growth with the injection of cell genes into the heart muscle; biomechanics, which has created the semi-automatic defibrillator and which will doubtless one day lead to the creation of a completely artificial heart. All of this knowledge and all these discoveries can only be improved upon.

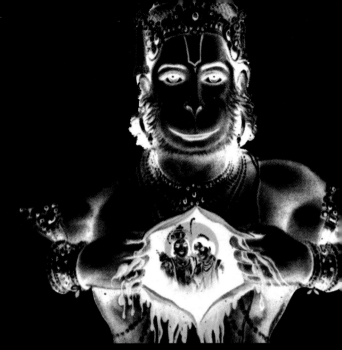

# LOOK

WHETHER ON GRAFFITI, SIGNS, LUCKY CHARMS, WALLS, MONUMENTS, TREES OR EVEN TATTOOED ON THE SKIN, THE HEART IS ON DISPLAY EVERYWHERE. THE FOLLOWING PAGES CONTAIN ARRESTING IMAGES SHOWING JUST HOW MUCH THE HEART HAS EMBEDDED ITSELF IN OUR PSYCHE.

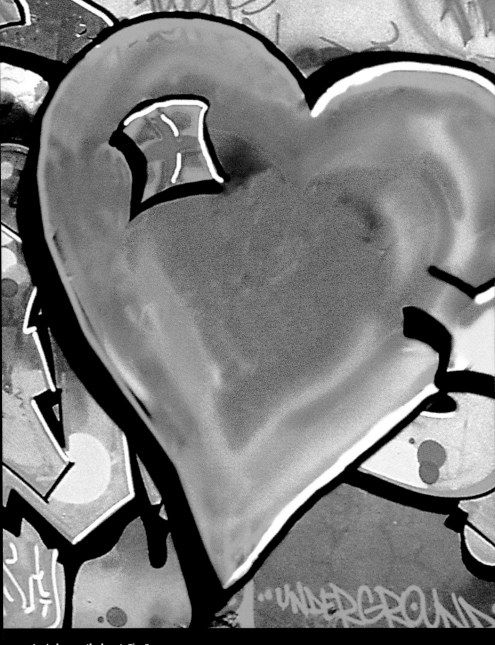

*A window on the heart.* The Bronx.

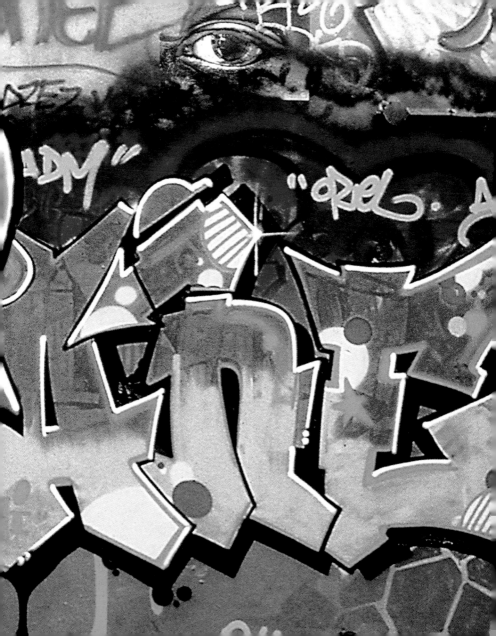

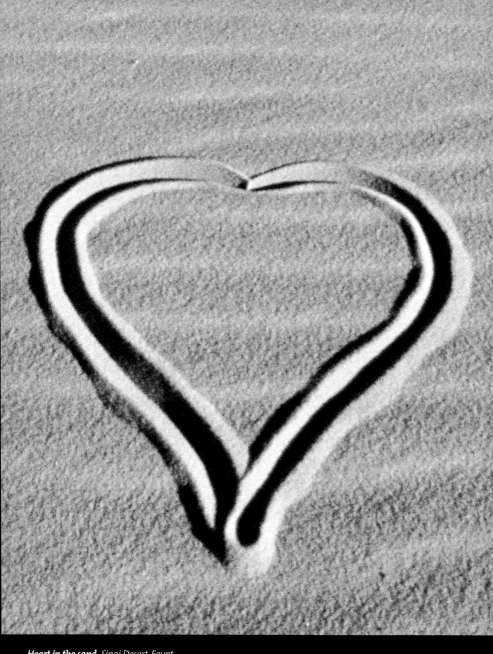

**Heart in the sand.** *Sinai Desert, Egypt.*

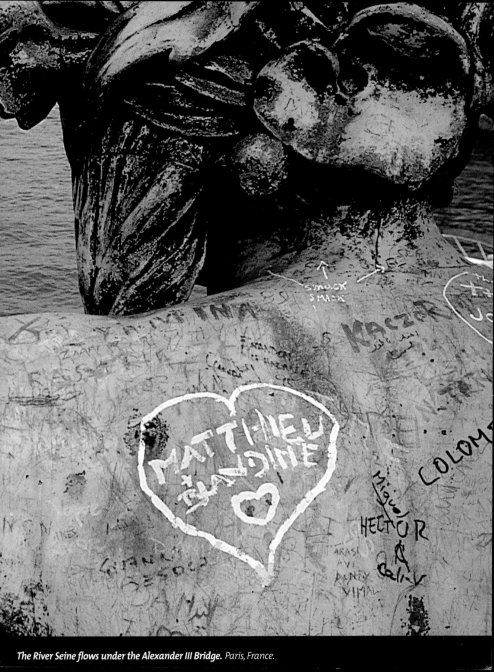

**The River Seine flows under the Alexander III Bridge.** *Paris, France.*

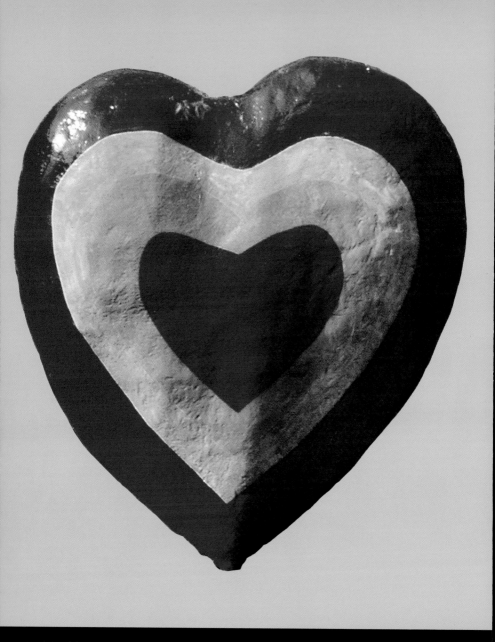

**Heart in celebration.** *Igor Stravinsky fountain, Nicky de Saint-Phalle (detail). Paris, France.*

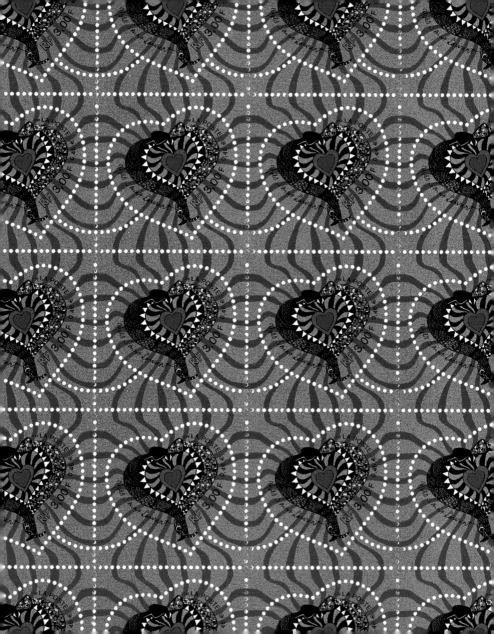

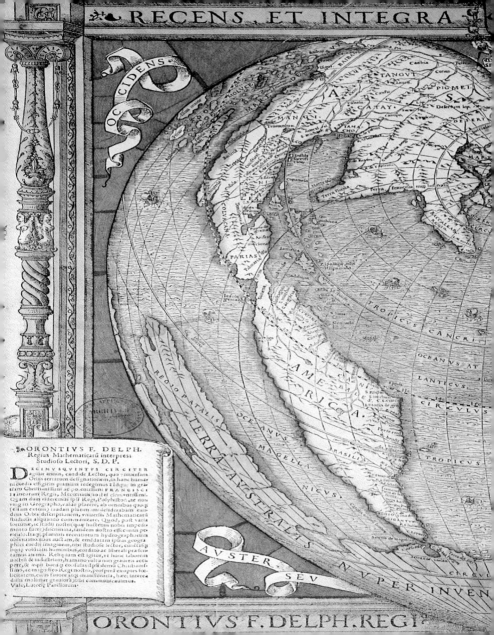

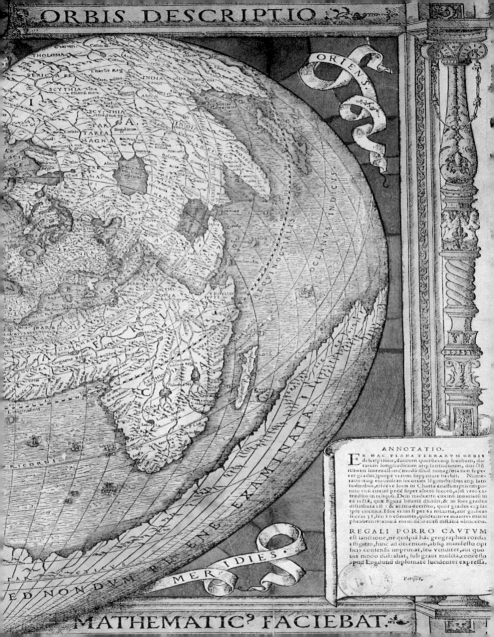

# ORBIS DESCRIPTIO

ORIENS

AEQVNOCTIALIS

OCEANVS INDICVS

SED NONDVM BENE EXAMINATA

MERIDIES

## ANNOTATIO.

EX HAC PLANA TERRARVM ORBIS
descriptione, duorum quorumcunque locorum, distarum longitudinum atque latitudinum, directum itinerus internallum, eo modo illud notagitur non superet gradus, ipsque verius sagittatae licebit. Numeratis itaque eorundem locorum longitudinibus atque latitudinibus, eisdéve locis in Charta coassumptis impono uno circini presse super altero locorum, ꝯ vero contedito in reliquu. Dein traducto circino insistati in ea recta, quae figura bifaria dividit, & in suos gradus distributa est: & animaduertito, quot gradus capiat ipse circuitus. Hos erum si per 24 multata, aut quolibet leucas 33 ad 60 communes, quidecunque maiore multiplicanti iratorú eorum de eo corú distátia obtinebu.

REGALI PORRO CAVTVM
est sanctione, ne quispiam hās geographici cordis effigiem, hinc ad decennium, absque manifesto opsficis consensu imprimat, seu venditet, aut quouis modo distrahat, sub graui multa, concesso apud Logdunü diplomate luculenter expressa.

Persiis.

## MATHEMATIC⁹ FACIEBAT.

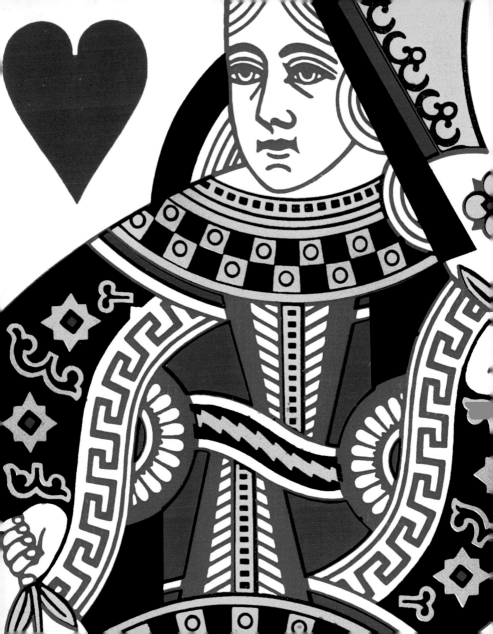

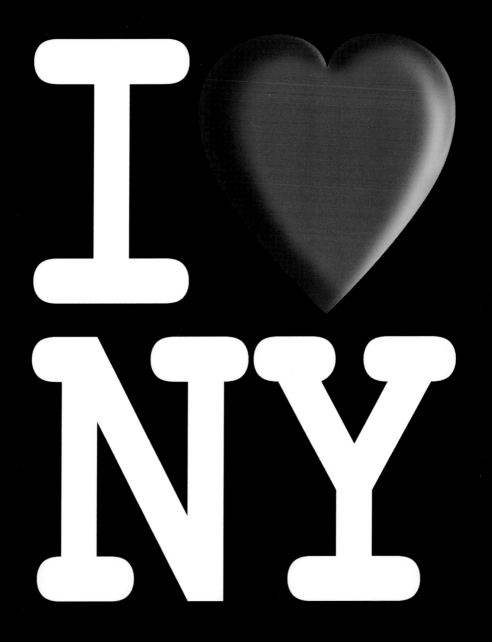

*Love in the heart of the city.*

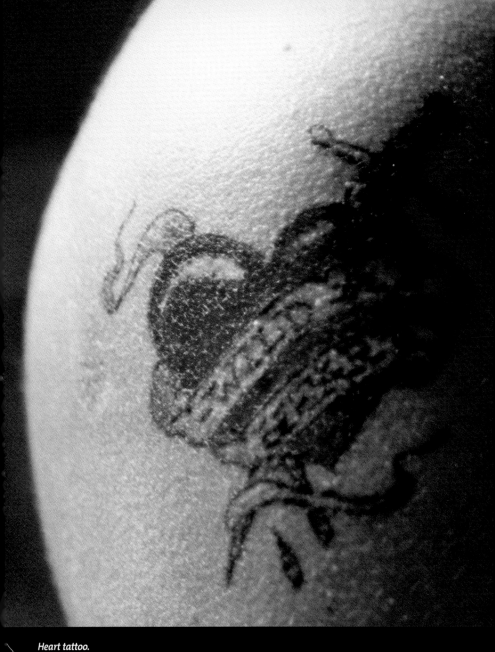

Heart tattoo.

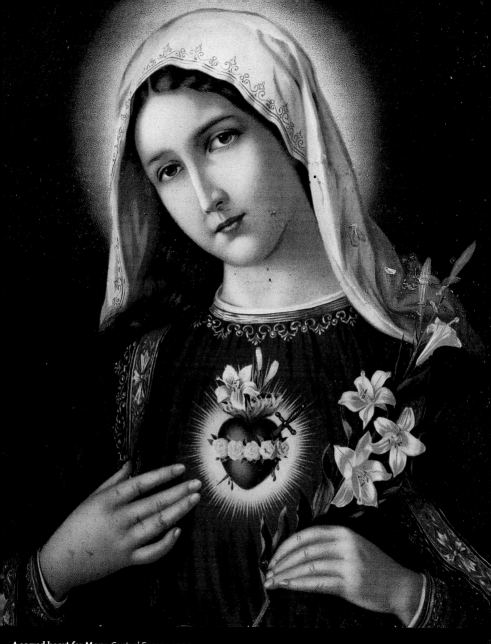

A sacred heart for Mary, Central Europe 1900

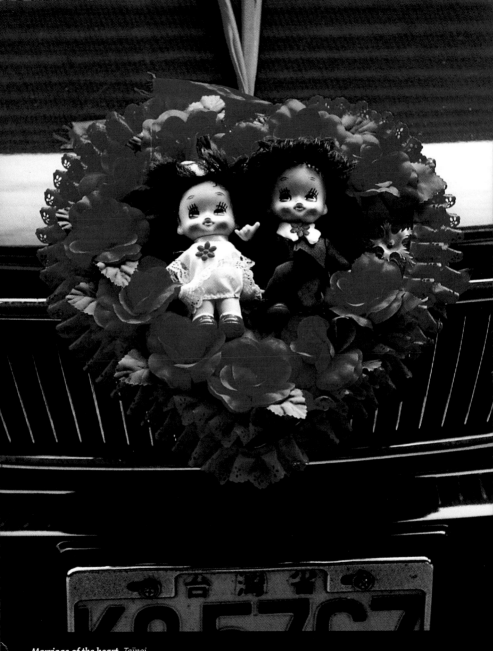

*Marriage of the heart, Tainai*

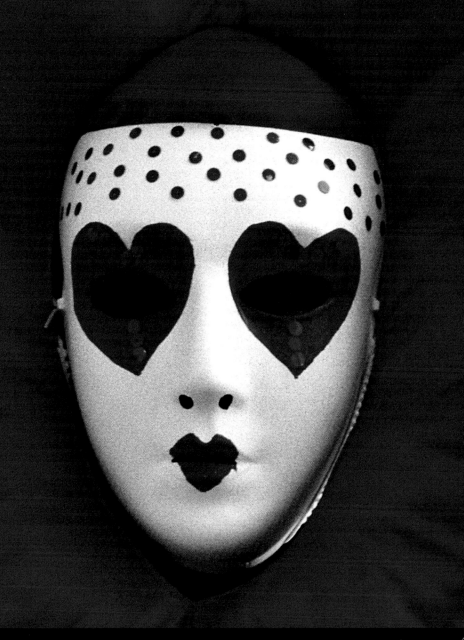

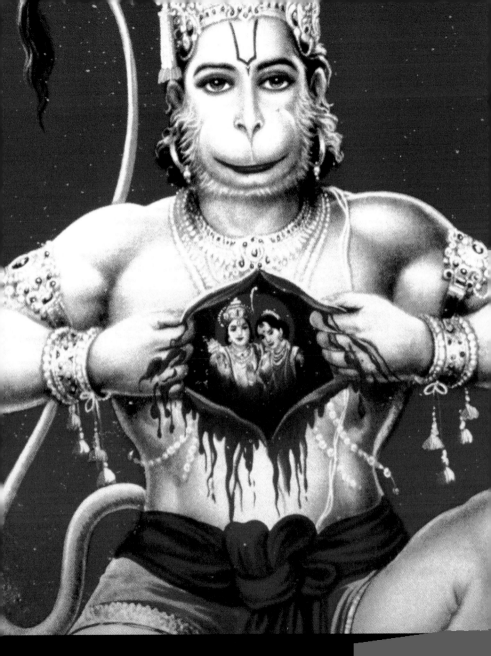

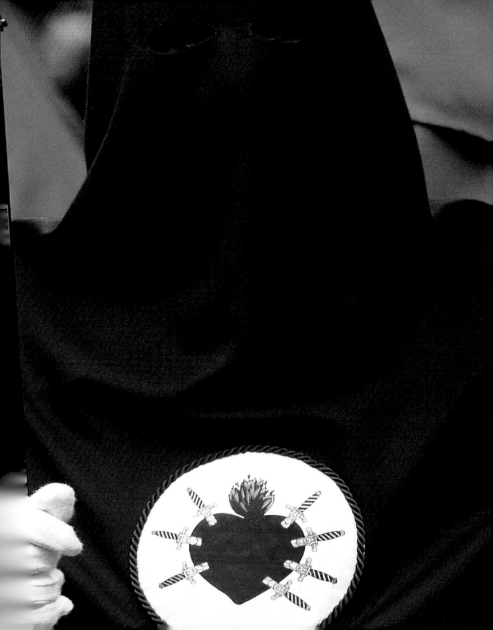

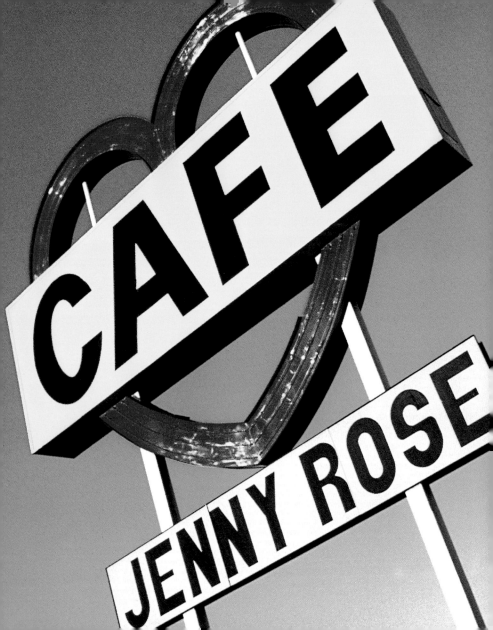

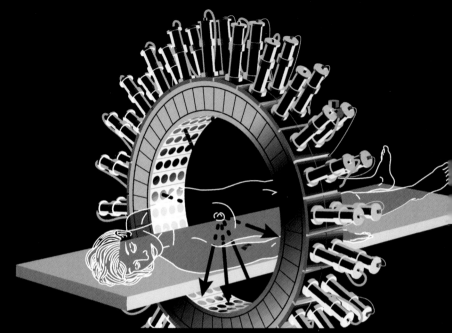

# IN PRACTICE

THE HEART IS AN INCREDIBLE PUMP THAT BEATS NON-STOP,
24 HOURS A DAY – HOW DOES IT WORK?
USING SOPHISTICATED MEDICAL IMAGING TECHNIQUES,
WE TAKE A JOURNEY INSIDE THE HEART AND ITS ARTERIES.
WE LOOK AT A SOUND, HEALTHY HEART AND
A DISEASED ONE IN NEED OF TREATMENT.

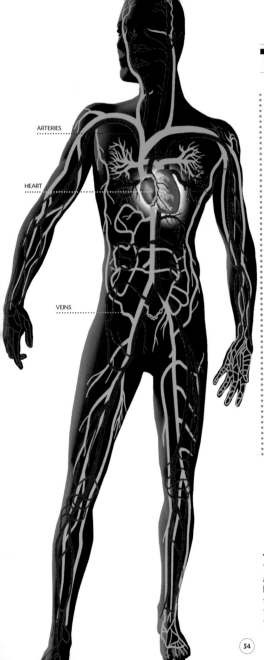

ARTERIES

HEART

VEINS

# The body's pump

**T**he heart sits between the two lungs, and is to the left of the centre of the thorax, surrounded by a fortress of bone and muscle.

### The heart revealed

The heart is a pump made of muscle. It contains cardiac cavities known as atria and ventricles. The atria receive blood and the ventricles expel it from the heart. The two largest blood vessels in the body extend out from the heart. The first is the aorta, the largest artery in our body, which comes out of the left ventricle, supplying oxygenated arterial blood to the whole body. The aorta supplies blood to the heart itself: the coronary arteries are vascular branches that stem from the root of the aorta.

The second is the vena cava, the largest vein in the body. The superior and inferior venae cavae return deoxygenated venous blood to the heart via the right atrium.

**THE BODY'S BLOOD CIRCULATION**
The heart is in the centre of the body; the veins are coloured blue, the arteries red. With each beat, the heart sends deoxygenated blood to the lungs, where it is oxygenated and returned to the heart before being transported throughout the body.

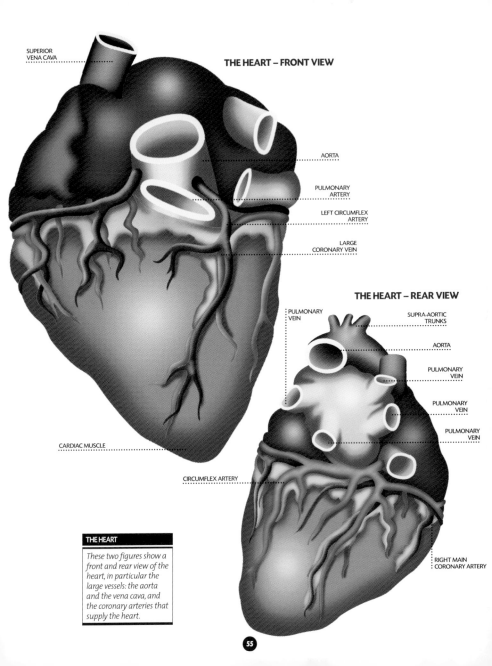

SUPERIOR
VENA CAVA

**THE HEART – FRONT VIEW**

AORTA

PULMONARY
ARTERY

LEFT CIRCUMFLEX
ARTERY

LARGE
CORONARY VEIN

**THE HEART – REAR VIEW**

PULMONARY
VEIN

SUPRA-AORTIC
TRUNKS

AORTA

PULMONARY
VEIN

PULMONARY
VEIN

PULMONARY
VEIN

CARDIAC MUSCLE

CIRCUMFLEX ARTERY

RIGHT MAIN
CORONARY ARTERY

**THE HEART**

*These two figures show a front and rear view of the heart, in particular the large vessels: the aorta and the vena cava, and the coronary arteries that supply the heart.*

# Inside the heart

The heart is divided in two by a wall of muscle, the septum. The right side of the heart collects blood from the body, while the left side collects blood from the lungs. The right and left sides are divided into two parts, each containing an atrium and a ventricle.

### The heart valves

These valves are very fine, supple, translucid membranes separating the atria from the ventricles. They have the vital function of ensuring that blood always flows from the atria to the ventricles. The valves work just like taps. When closed, they prevent any leakage of blood back from the way it came. When opened, they allow oxygenated blood to be pumped throughout the body and deoxygenated blood to be pumped to the lungs.

### The valves of the left side of the heart

The correct functioning of these valves (the mitral and aortic valves) is vital to the efficiency of the heart because the left side of the heart pumps blood at a much higher pressure than the right side in order to supply all of the body except the lungs. About nine or ten pints of blood are pumped out every minute.

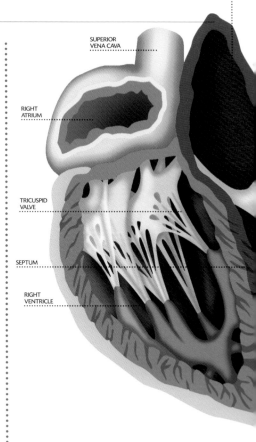

AORTA

SUPERIOR
VENA CAVA

RIGHT
ATRIUM

TRICUSPID
VALVE

SEPTUM

RIGHT
VENTRICLE

| ENDOSCOPY | |
|---|---|
| A probe equipped with an optical device is introduced into the patient's heart so that pictures of the heart valves can be displayed on a monitor. If the | valves are damaged, they can be repaired straight away. The technique used is known as valvuloplasty, a form of cosmetic surgery for heart valves. |

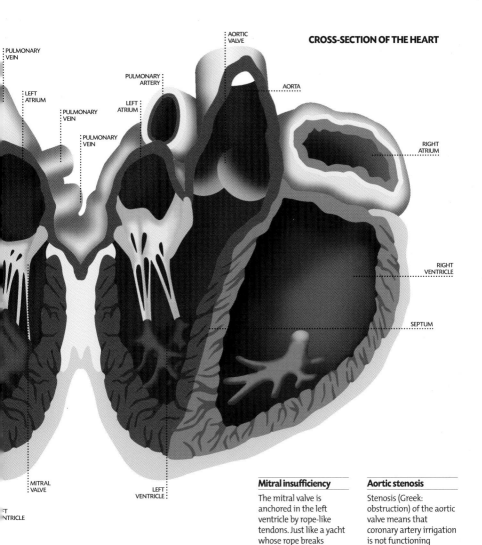

PULMONARY VEIN

LEFT ATRIUM

PULMONARY VEIN

PULMONARY VEIN

PULMONARY ARTERY

LEFT ATRIUM

AORTIC VALVE

AORTA

RIGHT ATRIUM

RIGHT VENTRICLE

SEPTUM

MITRAL VALVE

LEFT VENTRICLE

T NTRICLE

## Mitral insufficiency

The mitral valve is anchored in the left ventricle by rope-like tendons. Just like a yacht whose rope breaks during a storm, these tendons can be broken by a heart attack. The mitral valve is then said to escape.

## Aortic stenosis

Stenosis (Greek: obstruction) of the aortic valve means that coronary artery irrigation is not functioning properly. Aortic stenosis is one of the causes of coronary thrombosis and heart failure.

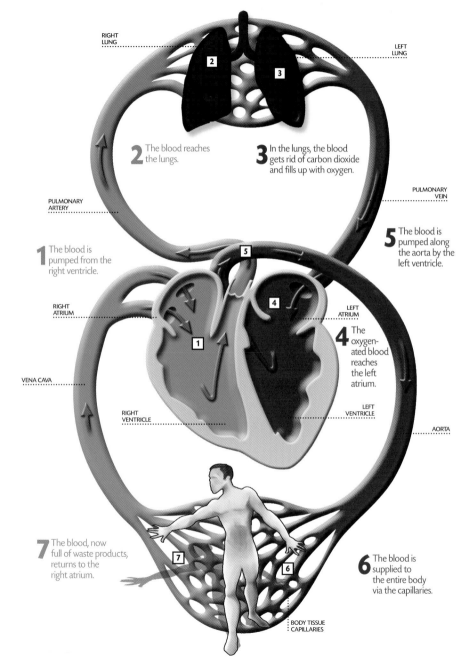

**RIGHT LUNG**

**2**

**3**

**LEFT LUNG**

**2** The blood reaches the lungs.

**3** In the lungs, the blood gets rid of carbon dioxide and fills up with oxygen.

**PULMONARY ARTERY**

**PULMONARY VEIN**

**5** The blood is pumped along the aorta by the left ventricle.

**1** The blood is pumped from the right ventricle.

**5**

**RIGHT ATRIUM**

**4**

**1**

**LEFT ATRIUM**

**4** The oxygenated blood reaches the left atrium.

**VENA CAVA**

**RIGHT VENTRICLE**

**LEFT VENTRICLE**

**AORTA**

**7** The blood, now full of waste products, returns to the right atrium.

**7**

**6**

**6** The blood is supplied to the entire body via the capillaries.

**BODY TISSUE CAPILLARIES**

# The vascular system: blood circulation

## The blood's journey around the body

Blood full of oxygen travels from the lungs along the pulmonary veins, then into the aorta, then distributed through the smaller arteries to the capillaries, which irrigate the body tissues. Here, the blood deposits its oxygen and collects carbon dioxide and waste matter. The venous circuit delivers the carbon dioxide-filled blood back to the vena cava, which transports it to the right atrium. From there, it is pumped by the right ventricle, via the pulmonary artery, towards the lungs, where it is reoxygenated.

### DANGER!

*If one of the coronary arteries is blocked by a coronary thrombosis, some heart cells die. This is a heart attack.*

The vascular system uses a double circuit to deliver blood, both to the organs according to their energy needs, and to the lungs.

## The different types of cells

The blood flowing inside the vessels contains three types of cells: white corpuscles, which fight against infection; red corpuscles, which carry oxygen; and, finally, platelets, which are responsible for blood clot formation. The most important blood cells in the context of heart disease are red corpuscles and platelets.

## Red corpuscles

These carry oxygen, which is vital to the heart muscle. If oxygen supply is reduced, the heart suffers and the pain of angina pectoris occurs. If the supply is stopped altogether, the heart muscle dies: this is a heart attack.

## Platelets

These are responsible for blood clotting. If a blood clot forms within a coronary artery it may affect blood flow to the heart muscle. In certain cases the clot, called a coronary thrombosis, may completely block the artery and so stop oxygen reaching the heart muscle.

## Arteries

Arteries are vessels that transport oxygenated blood (pictured in red) from the heart to the organs and body tissues. The exception is the pulmonary artery that carries deoxygenated blood from the heart to the lungs. The aorta is the largest of the arteries. It emerges from the left ventricle and transports oxygen-rich arterial blood throughout the body.

## Veins

Veins are vessels that return deoxygenated blood to the heart (pictured in blue). The exceptions are the pulmonary veins which carry oxygenated blood to the heart. The superior and inferior venae cavae return deoxygenated blood to the right atrium.

# The heart as a machine at work

**A** downward wave of electrical impulses over the heart controls the timing of heart contractions. The electrical stimulus passes over the atria first, making them contract, then over the ventricles.

### The automatic functioning of the heart
An electric current is created by a cluster of nerve cells, known as the sinoatrial node, sited in the right atrium. When heart rhythm is normal, ie regular, between 50 and 100 beats a minute, this is known as the sinus rhythm.

### Contraction of the atria
The current created in the sinoatrial node is conducted to the atria, which contracts pushing blood into the ventricles. The electrical impulse reaches the atrioventricular node, which is in the right atrium.

### Contraction of the ventricles
The impulse spreads through the wall of the ventricles, making them contract. Blood is pumped out into the body. During this phase, pressure in the blood vessels is high. The higher figure for blood pressure, systolic pressure, is measured at this point.

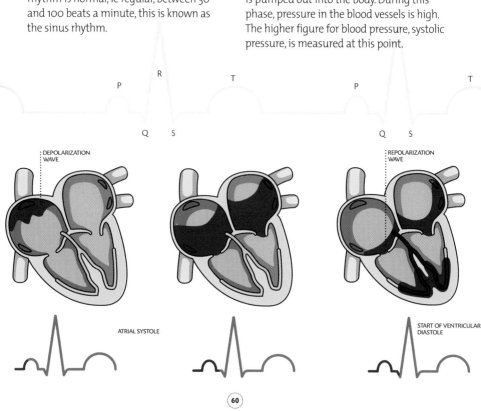

R

P

T

P

T

Q        S

Q        S

DEPOLARIZATION WAVE

REPOLARIZATION WAVE

ATRIAL SYSTOLE

START OF VENTRICULAR DIASTOLE

## Diastole (relaxation of the heart's muscle)

The heart relaxes and blood flows into the atria from the pulmonary veins and vena cava. At the end of diastole, the sinoatrial node generates another impulse.

## The electrocardiogram or ECG

Electric current travelling through the heart is picked up, so that an electrical map of the heart can be obtained. A normal trace contains small round positive waves (P), representing atrium contractions, and tall, narrow deflections (QRS), which represent ventricle contractions. The relaxation of the heart (diastole) is shown by wave T.

| WHEN THE IMPULSE NO LONGER GETS THROUGH | |
| --- | --- |
| In some cases, such as a heart attack, the heart's electrical activity is completely disorganized, causing ventricular fibrillation, a sort of short-circuit leading to cardiac and circulatory arrest. This is an extremely sudden and serious rhythm disorder. The ventricles do not contract and there is no | outflow from the heart. There is no blood supply to the brain, so the individual suddenly loses consciousness, producing an apparent state of death. Ventricular fibrillation is the most frequent cause of sudden death. However, it can be easily treated, using a defibrillator to administer an electric shock to the heart. |

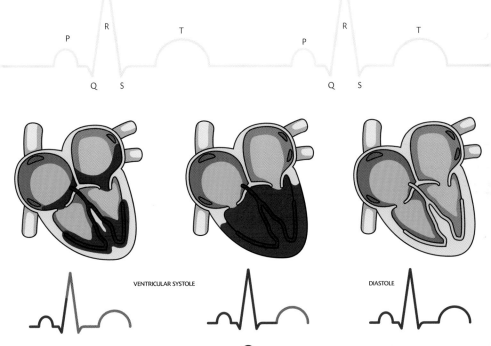

VENTRICULAR SYSTOLE

DIASTOLE

# The coronary arteries

Although they are very small (the largest have a diameter of 3 mm/0.1 inch, the smallest 0.5 to 1 mm/0.02 to 0.03 inch) the coronary arteries ensure the supply of oxygenated blood to the heart.

### A ring of arteries
The left and right coronary arteries emerge from two orifices in the aorta. They are arranged in a ring around the heart, hence their name (coronary = crown).

### The left coronary artery
This is the most important of the coronary arteries. The left ventricle works the hardest and has most need of oxygen to ensure the heart's output. The left ventricle is also the most likely to suffer from a coronary thrombosis (blockage) in its artery, the left coronary artery.

### Healthy arteries
In order to irrigate the heart properly, the coronary artery walls must be thin, supple, elastic and free from fatty, fibrous or calcium deposits.

### Plaques of atheroma
Atherosclerosis denotes degeneration of the arteries; the word comes from the Greek *scleros*, meaning 'hardening'. Plaques of atherosclerosis are deposits of cholesterol, calcium and fibrous tissue on the vascular wall.

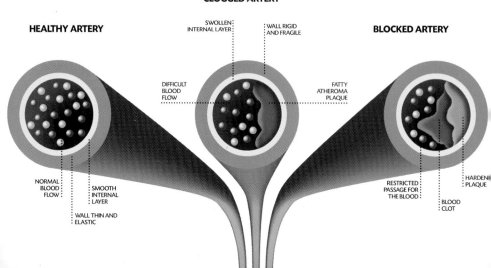

**CLOGGED ARTERY**

**HEALTHY ARTERY**

SWOLLEN INTERNAL LAYER

WALL RIGID AND FRAGILE

**BLOCKED ARTERY**

DIFFICULT BLOOD FLOW

FATTY ATHEROMA PLAQUE

NORMAL BLOOD FLOW

SMOOTH INTERNAL LAYER

WALL THIN AND ELASTIC

RESTRICTED PASSAGE FOR THE BLOOD

HARDENI PLAQUE

BLOOD CLOT

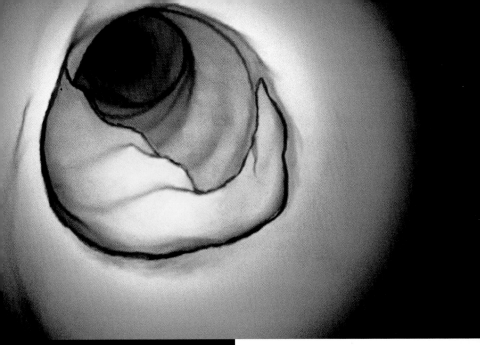

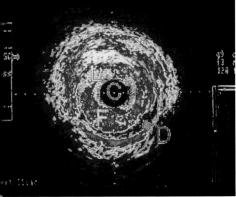

ABOVE, LARGE ATHEROMA PLAQUE (MORE THAN 35 PER CENT) AS SEEN BY A HELICAL ANGIOSCANNER.

BELOW, ENDO-ARTERIAL ULTRASOUND, ATHEROMA PLAQUE ADJOINING THE WALL OF THE LEFT INNER CAROTID, CONSIDERABLY REDUCING THE DIAMETER OF THE ARTERY. THE LETTERS ON THE PHOTOGRAPH CORRESPOND TO THE ATHEROMA PLAQUE (F), THE DIAMETER OF THE ARTERY (C), THE INNER CAROTID WALL (D) AND FATTY DEPOSITS (L).

## ATHEROSCLEROSIS: A LONG JOURNEY TOWARDS CORONARY THROMBOSIS

Atherosclerosis develops quietly and stealthily without visible symptoms for many years. But the partial obstruction of an artery prevents platelets – the tiny cells that make blood coagulate – from circulating freely. So they attach themselves to the fibrous mound and stimulate each other. A tough network of fibrin grows across the vascular opening. Very soon, this catches red corpuscles in its mesh and a blood clot or thrombosis forms. This can completely block the artery so that blood no longer circulates. A coronary thrombosis causes a heart attack. A thrombosis in the cerebral arteries causes cerebral vascular damage or stroke: a brain infarction.

# The symptoms of heart disease: pain and angina

A reduction of oxygen to the muscle of the heart causes the pain of angina pectoris (lack of oxygen to the heart). This often comes on after exertion but may also come on with increased emotion, cold weather, or following a meal. The reason for this is simple: the arteries are not completely blocked, and blood and oxygen are supplied in a quantity sufficient for a heart at rest. But once the heart's work-rate increases, its oxygen requirement increases as well. The obstructed artery can no longer keep up with the demand and the heart suffers.

## An attack of angina pectoris

Pain is felt beneath the left breast, like a tightening or powerful squeezing of the thorax. It may then spread, usually to the left arm, but also, and sometimes only, to the right arm. The sites of the pain vary, but is usually in the same place in a given individual: pain may be felt in the jaw, neck, back, wrists or hands.

Pain is sometimes felt as a mild discomfort in the chest, similar to indigestion. This may even be accompanied by cold sweats, palpitations, breathlessness, nausea or, more simply, overall fatigue or general discomfort.

These symptoms disappear after five or ten minutes' rest or, for people already diagnosed with angina pectoris, two to three minutes after taking a trinitroglycerin tablet or spray. Once exertion stops, the heart no longer needs extra oxygen. The blood supplied by the partially obstructed artery is, once again, sufficient; pain disappears after a short period of rest. If pain like this occurs for the first time, or if it persists, a doctor should be contacted immediately, as it may be due to a heart attack.

## Variant angina

The development of variant angina is unpredictable. It may occur in someone who did not previously suffer from angina, or it may occur in an angina sufferer who is already familiar with the symptoms. The individual feels more frequent or long-lasting pain, which may be more persistent than usual, or occur following exertion that the heart would normally cope with. It may even occur when the heart is at rest.

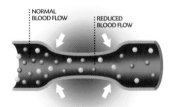

NORMAL BLOOD FLOW   REDUCED BLOOD FLOW

**CONTRACTED ARTERY**
During spastic angor, a type of variant angina with spasms, the artery contracts.

| CONDITIONS | EXAMPLES | REASONS |
|---|---|---|
| THE ENVIRONMENT | Smoking | Smoking increases heart rate, causes the arteries to constrict or close up (vasoconstriction) and decreases the level of oxygen in the blood. |
| | Heavy meals | Digestion increases the heart's work-rate. The stomach, intestine, liver and pancreas all need more energy, which comes to them via the blood and therefore the heart. |
| | Sexual activity | This increases heart rate and blood pressure. It causes the release of catecholamines (chemicals from the brain), which increase the heart's work-rate. |
| | Stress, anxiety, fear, anger, cold | All these similarly increase the heart's work, causing a rush of adrenaline. |
| | Exercise | Exercise increases the heart's work, and so in tests it is used for diagnosing angina. |
| ASSOCIATED DISEASES | Anaemia | This is a reduction in the number of red corpuscles, which transport oxygen. Anaemia therefore reduces the supply of oxygen to the heart. |
| | Fever | This increases heart rate. |
| | High blood pressure | In order to continue to irrigate all the organs, the heart has to fight against excessive vascular pressure. |
| MEDICINES | Cold remedies | Decongestants and anti-histamines increase heart rate. |
| | Drugs | Cocaine causes chest pain, which, in one third of cases, is a symptom of a genuine infarction, whatever the age of the individual. Amphetamines can cause very serious, even fatal, heart rate disorders. |
| | Terminating treatment for heart disease | Never terminate treatment for heart or blood pressure problems. Never stop taking aspirin, beta-blockers or anti-arrhythmics. |

# Heart attack

**M**yocardial infarction, or heart attack, is always serious and requires prompt treatment.

### What happens?
The problem is caused in one of two ways: either a plaque of atherosclerosis breaks off or is dislodged from the wall of a vessel supplying blood to the heart and suddenly obstructs the vessel, or a blood clot forms rapidly at the site of a plaque of atherosclerosis in a coronary artery, preventing blood from reaching the heart.

The heart muscle is no longer oxygenated and heart cells start to die. If the patient survives, the dead cells cannot be regenerated and heart muscle will be replaced by a fibrous scar tissue that cannot contract. If large areas of heart muscle are replaced by scar tissue, the heart cannot pump blood effectively.

### The unexpected heart attack
A heart attack can occur at any time, even during sleep, but most often early in the morning. It may be triggered by intensive exercise or a shock, and may occur without warning.

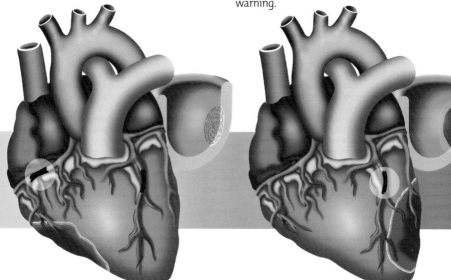

**LOWER HEART INFARCTION**
Because the obstruction is in the right coronary artery, a lower heart infarction has little effect on the strength of the heart's contraction. The outcome of this infarction is likely to be positive.

**LATERAL HEART INFARCTION**
Because of the obstruction to a branch of the left coronary artery, the circumflex artery, this type of infarction paralyses a large part of the left ventricle.

## Typical symptoms of a heart attack

A heart attack is characterised by pain similar to that in angina, accompanied by general fatigue, cold sweats, breathlessness, palpitations, nausea, vomiting, dizziness and, sometimes, loss of consciousness. The pain may be felt in several parts of the body: in the jaw, teeth, neck, left shoulder or middle of the back. The best thing to do is call for help and chew an aspirin tablet if one can be found.

## Highly deceptive symptoms

However, 20 per cent of heart attacks do not cause pain but, at worst, a temporary, unaccountable discomfort similar to indigestion. In addition, the intensity of the pain is not in proportion to the seriousness of the heart attack, hence one should never play down the symptoms felt. If there is any doubt, call for medical help immediately and chew an aspirin; every second counts.

## THE 1-2-3 AND ABC OF LIFESAVING

*First aid skills should be carried out correctly and not improvised. A single morning's training by St John's Ambulance or the Red Cross could help you learn these skills.*

*1-2-3: someone collapses.*
*1: Call for help by dialling 999.*
*2: Be assertive with the person. Try to find out if he has simply fainted or actually lost consciousness. Shout loudly, use his name, talk to him, tap him on the cheek or on the back, ask him how he's feeling.*

*3: Stay calm, whatever happens.*

*ABC: the person does not regain consciousness.*
*A: Airways. These must be open. Ensure that the chin is raised.*
*B: Breathing. Carry out two mouth-to-mouth resuscitations for every fifteen heart massages.*
*C: Circulation. Give heart massage by placing both palms on the sternum and pressing hard on the chest 80 to 100 times a minute.*

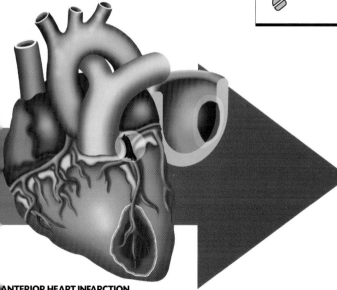

## Infarctions and scarring

The seriousness of an infarction is reflected by the size of the scar it leaves. Coronary thrombosis leaves the heart with irreversible cell death, which will be more or less widespread depending on the gravity of the infarction. This part of the heart will never contract again.

## ANTERIOR HEART INFARCTION

This is the most dangerous type of infarction. It is caused by obstruction of the front inter-ventricular artery, a branch of the left coronary artery, and will lead to the death of the front wall of the left ventricle, which is vital to the maintenance of good heart output.

# Complications accompanying heart attacks

A number of complications may accompany a heart attack, ranging from heart-rate disorders and cardiac insufficiency to blood clots, etc.

### Ventricular fibrillation (a serious heart rhythm disorder leading to almost immediate loss of consciousness)

With the blood supply interrupted, the heart cells suffocate, start to malfunction and are no longer able to transmit the nervous impulse that makes the heart muscle contract. But each heart fibre is still trying to do its work. Each receives its share of current, fibrillates and trembles, but is too weak to transmit the nerve impulse to its neighbour. The heart fibres cannot co-ordinate their contractions. The heart fails to pump effectively and stops pumping blood to the rest of the body. The brain is not supplied with oxygen, so the patient loses consciousness. The heart stops beating, the pulse ceases and death is imminent. Life can be saved only sometimes by an external electric shock from a defibrillator.

### A blood clot in the heart

When heart contractions are weak, blood can stagnate in the heart. Platelets then tend to form into clumps to create a blood clot. Alternatively, after recovery a clot may form around the fibrous scar tissue that replaces the area of dead heart muscle. When the heart beats, the clot may be pumped out into the circulatory system and cause what is known as an embolism. The clot lodges itself anywhere in the limbs, brain, or other organs, blocking the blood supply beyond it.

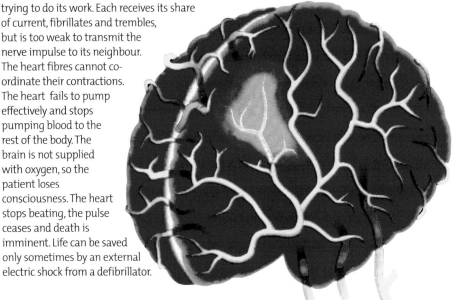

A STROKE, ONE OF THE COMPLICATIONS
CAUSED BY INFARCTION.

## COMPLICATIONS ACCOMPANYING INFARCTIONS

Cardiac arrest, heart fracture and cardiac insufficiency are all consequences of the death of part of the heart muscle.

### Oedemas and swelling of the legs

The right heart has difficulty in drawing in venous blood, which thus stagnates in the veins. These swell up as pressure in the vessels becomes too great. The liquid, known as plasma, in which red corpuscles circulate, is pushed by this pressure and passes through the vessel walls, infiltrating body tissues and creating oedemas. These are generally found in the legs, but occasionally in the stomach, when they are known as ascites.

### Heart aneurysm

Having suffered an infarction, the left ventricle wall bears a thin fibrous scar, which expands like a balloon outside the heart and may burst as a result of pressure. This is cardiac rupture – a rare cause of sudden death. Fortunately, such aneurysms are easily detected by an ultrasound scan, which is routinely carried out after any heart attack. It may be treated in time by an operation in which the weak tissue is removed and replaced, possibly even by one of the back muscles.

### Acute pulmonary oedema

Oxygenated blood in the lungs is not properly drawn in by the left side of the heart and starts to stagnate. As a result, pressure increases in the pulmonary blood vessels. Plasma passes through the vascular wall and infiltrates lung tissue. Within half an hour, the lungs may fill with water. The individual starts to feel breathless after the slightest exertion or even at rest. There should be no delay. Go straight to hospital at the first sign of breathlessness. Nowadays, excellent treatments are available, such as nitro compounds, diuretics and vasopressors that increase the strength of the heart. These take effect within seconds.

### Cardiac insufficiency

Following an infarction, the damaged part of the heart can no longer contract properly. The heart muscle cannot pump blood adequately through the body. Signs of cardiac insufficiency are general fatigue, breathlessness and, sometimes, acute pulmonary oedema.

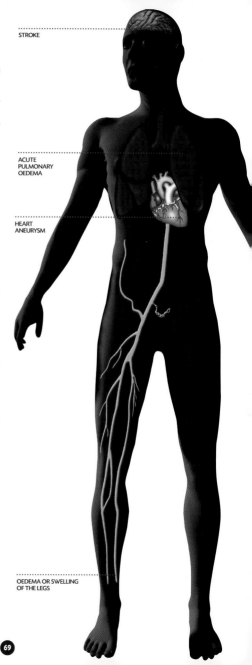

STROKE

ACUTE PULMONARY OEDEMA

HEART ANEURYSM

OEDEMA OR SWELLING OF THE LEGS

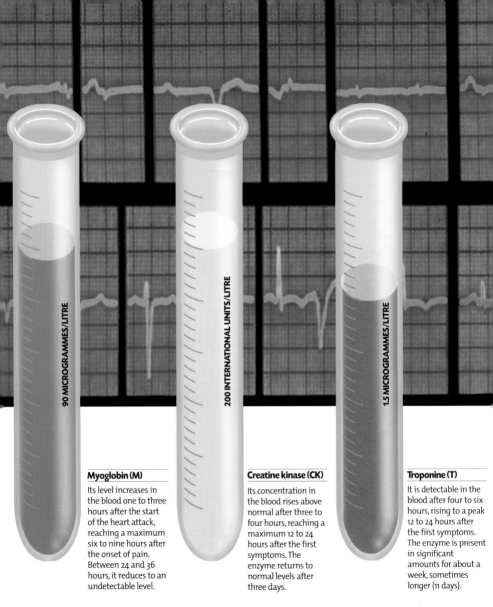

**90 MICROGRAMMES/LITRE**

**200 INTERNATIONAL UNITS/LITRE**

**1.5 MICROGRAMMES/LITRE**

### Myoglobin (M)

Its level increases in the blood one to three hours after the start of the heart attack, reaching a maximum six to nine hours after the onset of pain. Between 24 and 36 hours, it reduces to an undetectable level.

### Creatine kinase (CK)

Its concentration in the blood rises above normal after three to four hours, reaching a maximum 12 to 24 hours after the first symptoms. The enzyme returns to normal levels after three days.

### Troponine (T)

It is detectable in the blood after four to six hours, rising to a peak 12 to 24 hours after the first symptoms. The enzyme is present in significant amounts for about a week, sometimes longer (11 days).

# Diagnosing a heart attack

Every minute counts! If a doctor is faced with someone suffering acute chest pain, two tests will help determine whether the diagnosis is a heart attack: the electrocardiogram and the measurement of heart enzymes.

## The electrocardiogram (ECG) reads the heart's nervous impulses

The electrocardiogram reads the electric current passing through the heart and provides a detailed electrical map.

## The changes

In 90 per cent of cases changes are seen in the pattern of electrical impulses recorded by an ECG. Typically the 'ST' segment elevates above the line. Subsequently a new wave appears, dipping below the line (the Q-wave). Lastly, the T-wave, previously a peak above the baseline, becomes a valley or depression.

It is very important to be able to compare an electrocardiogram recorded at the time of the heart attack with a previous trace. Some individuals have an abnormal basic electrocardiogram, especially if they have already suffered a heart attack. It is therefore vital to know what changes have taken place in order to provide the most suitable treatment.

If you have had cause to have an electrocardiogram taken, try photocopying it, especially if it is abnormal, reducing it to the size of a credit card so that you can keep it in your wallet. In this way, should you need to seek advice from a doctor other than your own, for example in an emergency, the photocopied version might help the doctor to give a better diagnosis.

## A diagnosis via heart enzymes

During a heart attack, the dead heart cells release a number of enzymes and proteins into the blood, including some which are relatively specific for the heart muscle They include creatine kinase (CK) and its cardiac subunit, CK-MB, and two proteins, myoglobin and troponine. There is a detectable rise in these enzymes, released into the blood stream by the damaged heart muscle. If the pattern of this release is characteristic, it confirms that a heart attack has taken place.

---

**MOLECULES RELEASED DURING A HEART ATTACK: HEART ENZYMES AND PROTEINS**

*Three enzymes are essential to the diagnosis of an acute heart attack. So that they are not missed, several blood samples are taken at intervals of a few hours. For the same reason, if a heart attack is suspected, it is important to remain under observation for 24 hours.*

*Myoglobin (M)*
*Unfortunately, this is not very specific. It can be produced by any damaged muscle, and if the heart attack has occurred after physical exercise, it is not very helpful. However, it appears earlier than other molecules and, if there has been no muscular exertion,* *can point to a diagnosis of a heart attack within an hour or two of the appearance of symptoms.*

*Creatine kinase(CK)*
*CK-MB, a sub-unit of this enzyme, is specific to the heart.*

*Troponine (T)*
*The last of the heart proteins, troponine is very specific and sensitive, enabling doctors to diagnose very minor coronaries. With this protein, it is also possible to make a retrospective diagnosis of a heart attack as it stays in the blood for up to eleven days after the heart attack.*

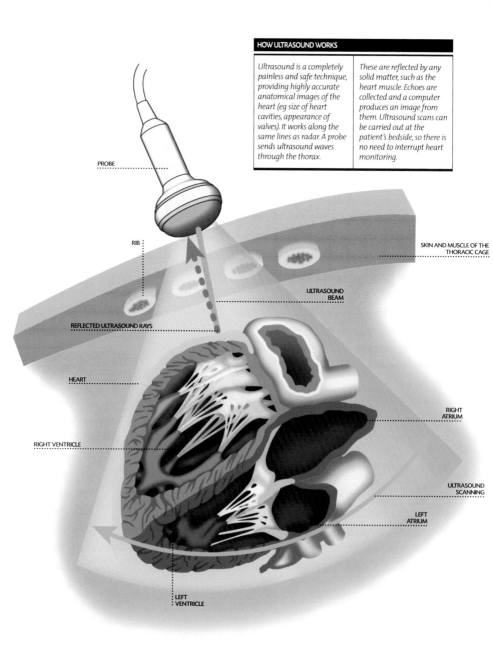

PROBE

RIB

SKIN AND MUSCLE OF THE
THORACIC CAGE

ULTRASOUND
BEAM

REFLECTED ULTRASOUND RAYS

HEART

RIGHT
ATRIUM

RIGHT VENTRICLE

ULTRASOUND
SCANNING

LEFT
ATRIUM

LEFT
VENTRICLE

# Exploring the coronary arteries

**E**chocardiograms and angiography are often carried out during the heart attack's acute phase and can enable doctors to treat the heart attack immediately via angioplasty (surgery to re-open blocked blood vessels). From the onset of the first symptoms, an ultrasound scan can be carried out at the patient's bedside. A period of observation and stabilisation is required before other methods of exploration can be brought into play.

### Heart ultrasound, or echocardiogram

Heart ultrasound can be very useful in diagnosing a heart attack when the electrocardiogram is not conclusive and the results of the enzyme test are not yet ready. In the case of a heart attack, the damaged area contracts badly or not at all. This is known as hypokinesia or akinesia (from the Greek *hypo*, little; *a*, without; and *kinesia*, movement). Heart ultrasound helps to trace this heart malfunction, which is a sure sign of a heart attack.

### An additional test

A specific type of ultrasound called Doppler Ultrasound Scanning is often carried out to observe blood flow in the heart and measure heart output. The test also enables doctors to check whether there is any flow of blood back from the left ventricle to the left atrium caused by mitral insufficiency.

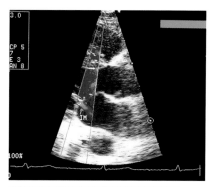

ULTRASOUND, COUPLED WITH A DOPPLER TEST, GIVES A COLOUR PICTURE OF THE MOVEMENT OF THE BLOOD THROUGH THE HEART CAVITIES.

### Trans-oesophageal ultrasound, another type of heart ultrasound

Trans-oesophageal ultrasound, or TOU, gives an almost direct view of the heart. Following local anaesthetic, a flexible plastic tube is passed through the mouth and into the oesophagus. From here, ultrasound waves have only to pass through the thin lining of the oesophagus wall to reach the heart and its valves. In this way, better pictures are obtained; the aorta can be examined and any blood clots in the ventricles are revealed, these are frequently one of the complications of myocardial infarction. An aneurysm in the aorta can also be spotted during TOU. Though not very pleasant, this test is quite safe and painless.

# The exertion test and scintigraphy

The exertion test reproduces the exertions of daily life, showing how the heart behaves when it has to work harder.

### Testing the heart at work

This gives an indirect view of the coronary arteries but may reveal coronary insufficiency, sometimes even before any symptoms have arisen. It is recommended as part of the screening process for patients at risk, when an anomaly is spotted on the basic electrocardiogram or if symptoms similar to angina pectoris occur during exertion. It is also prescribed following a heart attack, as a check to make sure that the heart is not suffering and that medication is effective.

For patients who are bed-ridden or unable to do any exercise prior to an operation, drugs are used to artificially increase the heart's work-rate. Doctors also carry out heart ultrasound and scintigraphy alongside this test.

**EXERTION TESTS**

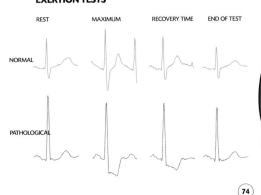

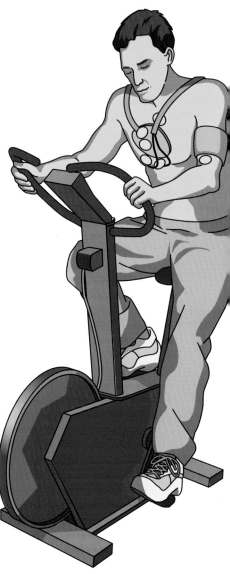

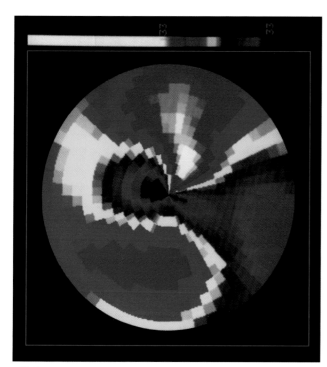

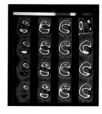

MYOCARDIAL SCINTIGRAPHY SHOWING AN AREA OF ISCHAEMIA OR NECROSIS. THE DAMAGED AREA PICKS UP THE MARKER LESS WELL, GIVING A DIFFERENCE IN COLOURING.

### Is this test risky?

The exertion test involves risk, but this is rare and controllable. What the cardiologist is trying to show, and indeed induce, is heart ischaemia (inadequate blood flow). By reproducing the conditions likely to cause ischaemia, it is possible that an attack of angina pectoris, heart rate disorders and even, rarely, a heart attack might be triggered. If this does happen, it should not be regarded as a mistake on the part of the doctor. In this case, the ischaemia would have occurred anyway, unexpectedly and without the presence of a cardiologist ready to stabilise and treat this type of situation. In fact, an exertion test could save a patient's life.

### Scintigraphy

When carried out together with an exertion test, this test gives more detailed information about the coronary arteries.

Scintigraphy shows how blood moves through the blood vessels and chambers of the heart. A radioactive substance is injected into the bloodstream and is picked up in different amounts by different tissues. The substance gives off radiation that is picked up by a camera to produce a digitalised image on a screen. Technetium is the most widely used marker. More of it is taken up by the well-supplied heart cells, thus enabling doctors to identify the darker areas where the heart attack has occurred.

### What is it like to have scintigraphy?

The exertion test combined with technetium scintigraphy is painless, though hard work! It is performed like an x-ray, the quantity of radiation emitted is negligible, but it is more sensitive at detecting ischaemia than a simple exertion test.

Images are produced straight after exertion and again two to four hours later; this corresponds to the revascularisation time required if the coronary arteries are defective. The test may be carried out as soon as the patient is admitted to casualty. A large number of patients complain of chest pain, even though their electrocardiogram is normal. Scintigraphy may help in this situation, but is not done routinely in the UK. Usually an exercise ECG and echocardiogram supply all the information about your heart that doctors need.

# Using coronary angiography for a live picture of the coronary arteries

**A**ngiography – literally, an X-ray of the coronary arteries – provides a picture of the arteries that supply the heart, using a radio-opaque contrast substance.

### A picture of the coronary arteries

Virtually painless and almost completely safe (less than 0.1 per cent complication rate), it is the most used, most accurate, most reliable and most direct method of providing a picture of the coronary arteries.

It enables the cardiologist to spot shrinkage of as little as 1 or 2 mm/0.05 inch and to see whether collateral circulation has formed, where tiny vessels are created to bypass an obstacle in a coronary artery.

In this way, the cardiologist can assess the condition of the coronary arteries and determine the most appropriate form of treatment for each patient (angioplasty, coronary bypass or drugs). Angiography can thus prevent heart attacks and save lives.

### What happens after angiography?

Angioplasty can be carried out immediately during angiography. If a coronary bypass is required, it can be scheduled to take place a few days later.

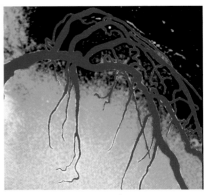

ICORONARY ANGIOGRAPHY IMAGE OBTAINED BY COMPUTERIZED DIGITAL ABSTRACTION. THE PROGRESS OF THE RADIO-OPAQUE SUBSTANCE IS UNINTERRUPTED. THERE IS NO SIGN OF OBSTRUCTION TO THE CORONARY ARTERY.

### RISKS ASSOCIATED WITH CORONAROGRAPHY

The injected contrast substance may cause an allergy. But this risk is easily identifiable and can be averted by antihistamines. Cardiac risks are very rare. The positioning of the catheter inside the coronary arteries may cause irritation to the heart. The heartbeat may become temporarily irregular. In rare cases, the catheter causes irritation in the coronary arteries, and a slight spasm leads to brief heart ischaemia. For an experienced doctor, these complications are easy to treat. The medical team should be made up of cardiologists who carry out this test several times a day and can anticipate all eventualities. The hospital should be a specialist centre with operating theatres and intensive care rooms available throughout the test.

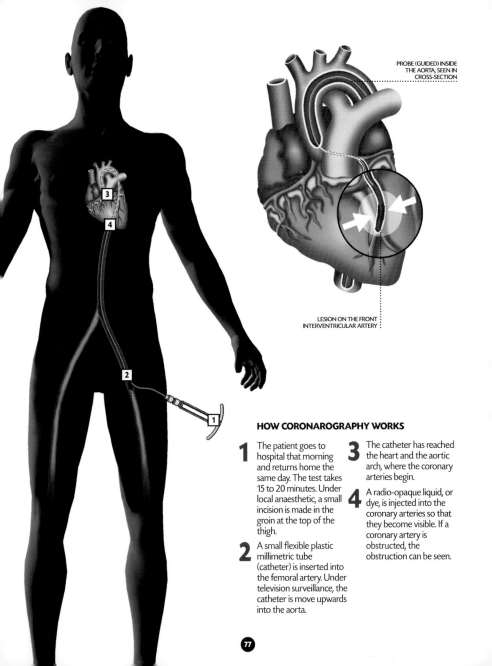

PROBE (GUIDED) INSIDE THE AORTA, SEEN IN CROSS-SECTION

LESION ON THE FRONT INTERVENTRICULAR ARTERY

## HOW CORONAROGRAPHY WORKS

**1** The patient goes to hospital that morning and returns home the same day. The test takes 15 to 20 minutes. Under local anaesthetic, a small incision is made in the groin at the top of the thigh.

**2** A small flexible plastic millimetric tube (catheter) is inserted into the femoral artery. Under television surveillance, the catheter is move upwards into the aorta.

**3** The catheter has reached the heart and the aortic arch, where the coronary arteries begin.

**4** A radio-opaque liquid, or dye, is injected into the coronary arteries so that they become visible. If a coronary artery is obstructed, the obstruction can be seen.

# Drugs for the heart

## Quick acting

Trinitroglycerin, a derivative of nitroglycerin in the form of a tablet that dissolves under the tongue for faster effect, is capable of dilating the coronary arteries in just a few minutes. It is a vasodilator, enabling blood to circulate more easily by widening the vessels through which the blood must pass. Trinitroglycerin is also available as a patch or a spray.

## Calcium channel blockers

These block the transport of calcium in the heart and blood vessel cells, thereby causing the muscle in the walls of these vessels to relax and increasing the diameter of the coronary arteries, reducing blood pressure. Diltiazem is one of the common channel-blockers to be used.

## Beta-blockers

Beta receptors are found on the membranes of heart cells. When stimulated by adrenaline or noradrenaline, they cause the heart to beat faster. Beta-blockers therefore slow and regulate the heart, and also reduce blood pressure. Even if the patient is involved in intense physical exercise, the heart rate remains slow and blood pressure low. Thus, beta-blockers protect the heart against any sudden excessive workload or any increased oxygen demand that obstructed coronary arteries could not satisfy. They are prescribed after a heart attack in order to prevent a relapse.

**T**hrombolysis and angioplasty are the emergency treatments for a heart attack. Nowadays, thanks to the emergency medical services and progress in resuscitation techniques, they are available to everyone.

## Thrombolytics: the hit squad

Thrombolysis is currently one of the best medical treatments for coronary thrombosis. It consists of dissolving the blood clot and preventing it from spreading through an intravenous injection of specific enzymes known as thrombolytics, which were discovered in the 1980s. These drugs are spectacularly effective, dissolving the blood clot so that the obstruction disappears from the electrocardiogram in only 15–20 minutes. Some people, however, may not be able to receive these drugs due to other medical conditions.

## A race against time

Time is in fact the main limiting factor. If these drugs are administered more than six hours after symptoms have started, they are much less effective. It is therefore essential to get to hospital quickly if an infarction is to be avoided. However, because they decrease the blood's ability to clot, thrombolytics increase the risk of a haemorrhage.

### ASPIRIN: A GREAT DEFENCE AGAINST HEART ATTACKS

At the first appearance of symptoms, the patient is given aspirin to dissolve under the tongue. The aspirin is thus absorbed immediately into the circulatory system, acting swiftly to paralyse platelets and prevent clot formation. A large number of studies have proved its effectiveness. It has been demonstrated that aspirin is even more effective than thrombolytic drugs.

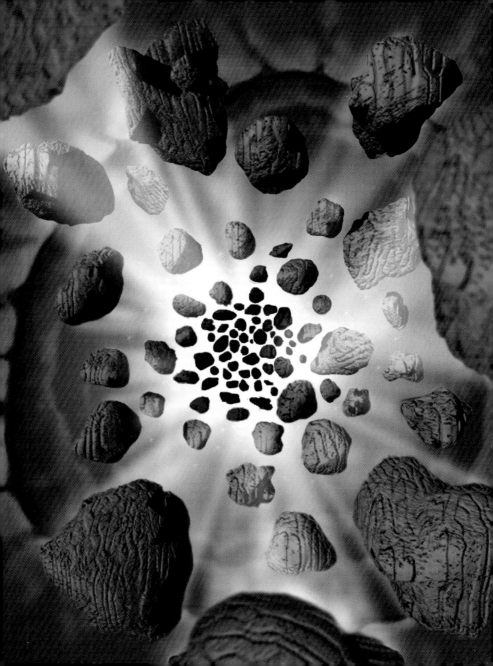

# New heart imaging techniques

**I**n recent years there has been considerable progress in medical imaging. Scanners and MRIs are inceasingly efficient, allowing cardiologists to observe the structure of the heart and the interior of the coronary arteries.

### Magnetic resonance imaging (MRI)

3-D MRI reveals atheroma plaques before they start to affect the arteries. Atherosclerosis can therefore be treated very early and heart attacks can be avoided through the use of new drugs such as statins and 'super-aspirins'.

### How MRI works

MRI images are obtained by placing a magnetic field around the body. This magnetic field makes atoms vibrate. The vibrations are captured and reconstituted by a computer. The procedure is painless, but the patient has to spend an hour in the MRI chamber.

MAGNETIC RESONANCE IMAGING

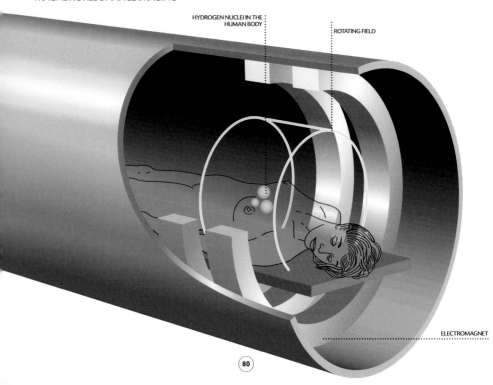

HYDROGEN NUCLEI IN THE HUMAN BODY

ROTATING FIELD

ELECTROMAGNET

# THE SCANNER

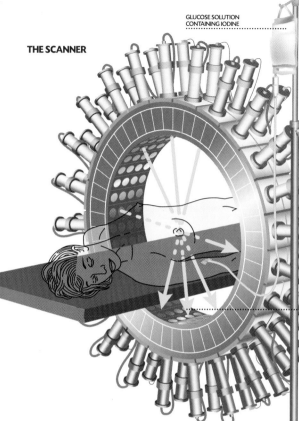

GLUCOSE SOLUTION
CONTAINING IODINE

SLIDING
TABLE

GAMMA RAY
DETECTORS

GAMMA RAY
EMISSIONS

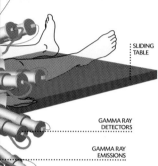

## The scanner

This radiographic technique is less accurate than MRI. However, a helical angioscanner is currently being developed that is likely to compare very favourably with 3-D MRI.

## INFRA-RED FIBRE OPTICS

We now know that the danger of atheroma plaques stems not from their size but from their instability. The sudden obstruction of the coronary arteries is often caused by the disintegration or rupture of the plaque. Having demonstrated that an unstable atheroma plaque was warmer than a stable plaque because of its inflammatory nature, researchers have succeeded in measuring intracoronary temperature, using infra-red fibre optics introduced into the coronary arteries. This technique is still in its early stages.

## The advantages of the scanner

Though older than MRI, it is better known and better understood. In addition, and unlike MRI, it can be used on patients equipped with old-fashioned (metal) heart valves or pacemakers.

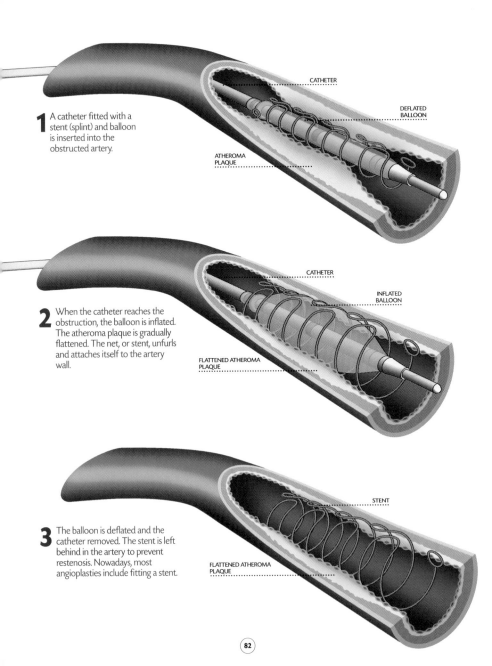

**CATHETER**

**DEFLATED BALLOON**

**ATHEROMA PLAQUE**

**1** A catheter fitted with a stent (splint) and balloon is inserted into the obstructed artery.

**CATHETER**

**INFLATED BALLOON**

**FLATTENED ATHEROMA PLAQUE**

**2** When the catheter reaches the obstruction, the balloon is inflated. The atheroma plaque is gradually flattened. The net, or stent, unfurls and attaches itself to the artery wall.

**STENT**

**FLATTENED ATHEROMA PLAQUE**

**3** The balloon is deflated and the catheter removed. The stent is left behind in the artery to prevent restenosis. Nowadays, most angioplasties include fitting a stent.

# Repairing coronary arteries

**A**ngioplasty was first carried out in Switzerland in 1977. A form of plastic surgery for the arteries, the principle is simple.

## How angioplasty works

Angioplasty involves inserting a balloon in the obstructed part of the coronary artery and then inflating the balloon to flatten the obstruction and push the artery walls apart. Blood can therefore start to flow again and reach the heart to supply it with oxygen.

It appears that angioplasty is currently the best treatment for a heart attack. It is more effective than anticoagulants and does not entail the risk of haemorrhage.

## How is angioplasty carried out?

The procedure starts with an angiogram. A probe fitted with a balloon is introduced into the femoral artery via an incision in the thigh. It is then moved up to the coronary arteries. A substance that contrasts with the blood is injected into the arteries so that the coronary artery obstruction can be seen by X-ray. The balloon can thus be correctly positioned and inflated. The obstruction remains but it is much smaller. The balloon is then removed. The patient remains conscious throughout the procedure and only a local anaesthetic is needed.

## Restenosis

The most frequent complication after angioplasty is recurring obstruction (restenosis) of the artery. When the balloon is used, the chances of the artery blocking again within six months are around 30 per cent.

In addition, the artery is sometimes blocked by a plaque of hard calcium that the balloon cannot crush. It has therefore been necessary to find other solutions, such as the stent, rotablator, extractor and even laser. The latter is used inside the coronary arteries, even though they may only be a few millimetres in diameter, to burn and remove debris. The rotablator – a rotating metal ball – eats away the calcified obstruction and the extractor is made of rotating blades that chisel away and remove hard plaque. The stent is a tiny wire mesh tube left in the artery to keep a clear passage.

## Avoiding restenosis

Anti-plaque drugs must be taken regularly. If the patient stops taking these drugs without medical advice, the coronary arteries may become obstructed again.

## Is it a dangerous operation?

Angioplasty saves thousands of lives every day. However, there is a risk of infarction: for a brief moment, when the balloon is inflated, the artery is completely blocked. This is a very rare occurrence, even rarer if a stent is used.

However, if it occurs, experienced cardiologists are always on hand to intervene immediately.

## What if it fails?

Angioplasty is recommended for most heart attacks. At present it is clearly one of the best treatments. However, if medical treatment has failed and angioplasty has not succeeded in unblocking the artery, then an operation is often required. For this reason, a surgical team is always on stand-by when an angioplasty is carried out.

Coronary bypass is now a very common operation and much safer than it used to be.

# Heart operations

The coronary bypass is one of the commonest operations undertaken in cardiology. In the hands of an experienced surgeon, the chances of full recovery are very high. It can be carried out as an emergency procedure after a heart attack, but is more often scheduled following coronarography.

The most common heart operation is the coronary artery bypass. A minimally-invasive procedure for this operation has now been developed.

## Minimally-invasive bypass but maximum progress

This is still a relatively uncommon procedure. However, the benefits suggest it is likely to become much more widespread in future. An incision is made on one side of the patient's thorax. A small artery in the thorax, called a mammary artery, is taken out to be used as a graft. A probe with a light source, called an endoscope, is inserted into the skin incisions. Guided by television pictures from the endoscope, the surgeon sutures the graft on to a branch of the aorta and then below the obstacle in the coronary artery.

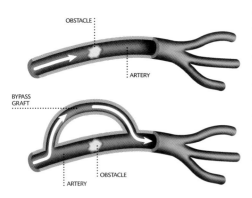

OBSTACLE

ARTERY

BYPASS GRAFT

OBSTACLE

ARTERY

## The graft

The mammary artery is much more suitable than the saphena vein as graft material. Patients who have had recurring obstructions have survived for an average of 10 years after a bypass using a saphena vein and 20 years after mini-invasive surgery using a mammary artery.

| | STANDARD CORONARY BYPASS | MINI-INVASIVE SURGERY |
|---|---|---|
| NUMBER OF ARTERIES BYPASSED | up to 5 | up to 2 |
| SCARS | 2 large ones (on the sternum and the leg) | one 10 cm/4 in long under the left breast; also under the right breast if two grafts are used |
| STERNUM | open | not affected |
| CARDIOPULMONARY BYPASS | necessary | unnecessary |
| HOSPITALIZATION | about 10 days | about 5 days |

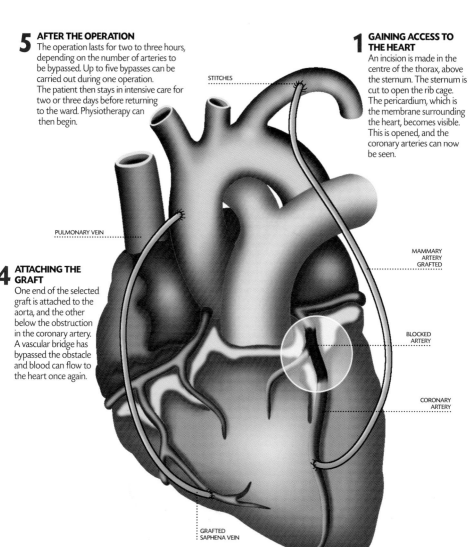

**5 AFTER THE OPERATION**
The operation lasts for two to three hours, depending on the number of arteries to be bypassed. Up to five bypasses can be carried out during one operation. The patient then stays in intensive care for two or three days before returning to the ward. Physiotherapy can then begin.

STITCHES

**1 GAINING ACCESS TO THE HEART**
An incision is made in the centre of the thorax, above the sternum. The sternum is cut to open the rib cage. The pericardium, which is the membrane surrounding the heart, becomes visible. This is opened, and the coronary arteries can now be seen.

PULMONARY VEIN

MAMMARY ARTERY GRAFTED

**4 ATTACHING THE GRAFT**
One end of the selected graft is attached to the aorta, and the other below the obstruction in the coronary artery. A vascular bridge has bypassed the obstacle and blood can flow to the heart once again.

BLOCKED ARTERY

CORONARY ARTERY

GRAFTED SAPHENA VEIN

**3 STOPPING THE HEART**
As it is very difficult to operate on a beating heart, a procedure known as cardiopulmonary bypass is used. While the graft is put in place, a heart-lung machine takes over the heart's job.

**2 PREPARING THE GRAFT**
Meanwhile, another surgeon is preparing the graft. The saphena vein from the leg and the mammary artery can be used.

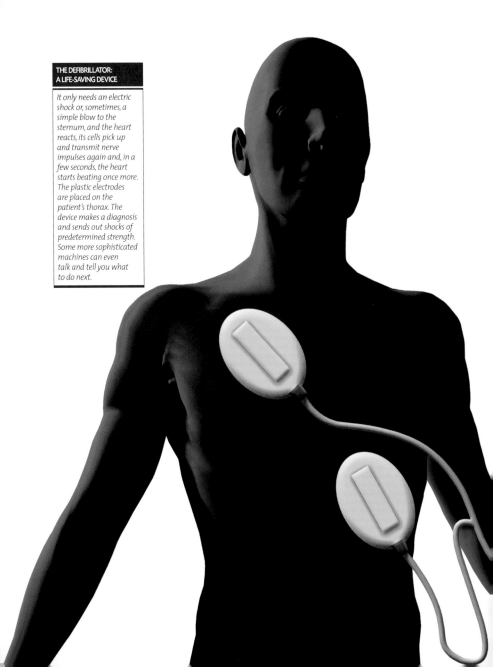

# Pacemakers and defibrillators

## The defibrillator implant

Miniaturization has led to the design of small defibrillators. These are implanted under the skin and can identify fibrillation, a heart rhythm disorder in which the heart stops beating. The devices react automatically, delivering a painless electric shock. If the first shock is ineffective, they deliver more. If the heart still does not start beating, they can act as a pacemaker (stimulator).

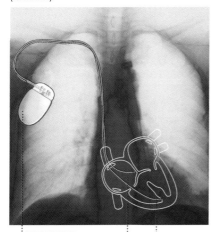

DOUBLE-CHAMBER
PACEMAKER WITH TWO
PROBES, ONE GOING TO
THE RIGHT ATRIUM, THE
OTHER TO THE TIP OF
THE RIGHT VENTRICLE.

RIGHT
ATRIUM

RIGHT
VENTRICLE

The implantable defibrillator saves many lives every day. Using these devices has reduced deaths from all kinds of abnormalities of the cardiac rhythm. They are more effective than any drugs currently in use.

## The ventricular assistant

This device supports the heart of an individual suffering from severe cardiac insufficiency who is waiting for a graft. It enables the patient to maintain a good quality of life.

It is implanted below the abdomen and helps the overworked left ventricle to pump blood into the aorta. In practice, blood is diverted from the left ventricle towards the device from where it is pumped forcibly into the aorta. This technology is still experimental and not routinely used in the UK.

## The pacemaker, an efficient timekeeper

Modern pacemakers work on demand, sending an electrical impulse only when the heart rate is too slow or a beat is missed. They increase heart rate automatically, just as the heart should do when we exert ourselves physically and breathe faster.

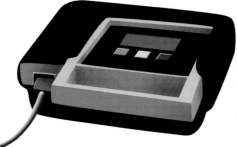

### The semi-automatic defibrillator

Thanks to a computer, this is always ready to diagnose and treat cardiac arrest. It is said to be idiot-proof, in that it is very simple to use.

# The artificial heart

This is every bio-technician's dream. Its aim is to reproduce the beating of the heart, but it is a very tall order to design a machine that will never break down. The patient's life will depend solely on how well this mechanical pump works.

## The transplant, a step on the way to the artificial heart

The first heart transplant took place more than 30 years ago in South Africa by Dr Christiaan Barnard. The operating technique is now well perfected, but it suffers from a crucial lack of donors, and touches on a fundamental question of ethics: the life of a patient depends on the death of another individual, whose heart (and soul?) is going to be removed and transplanted into an unknown person. This is also one of the reasons why doctors have recoursed to xenografting, in which damaged human heart valves are often replaced by the heart valves of calves or pigs. These animal heart valves are tolerated by the human body and, unlike metal heart valves, do not require the patient to take anticoagulants for life.

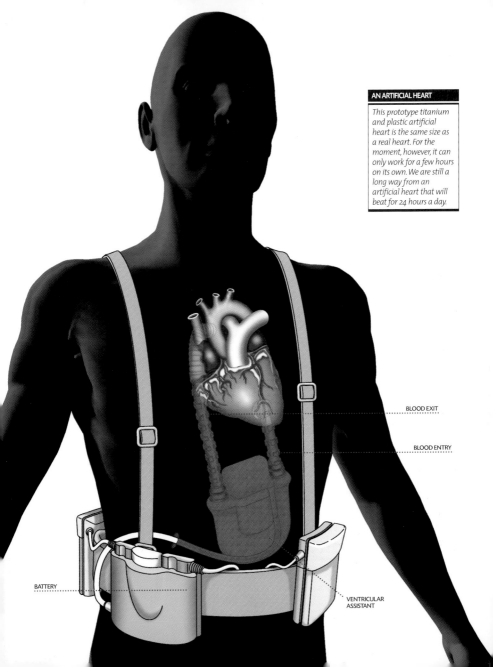

**AN ARTIFICIAL HEART**

*This prototype titanium and plastic artificial heart is the same size as a real heart. For the moment, however, it can only work for a few hours on its own. We are still a long way from an artificial heart that will beat for 24 hours a day.*

BLOOD EXIT

BLOOD ENTRY

BATTERY

VENTRICULAR ASSISTANT

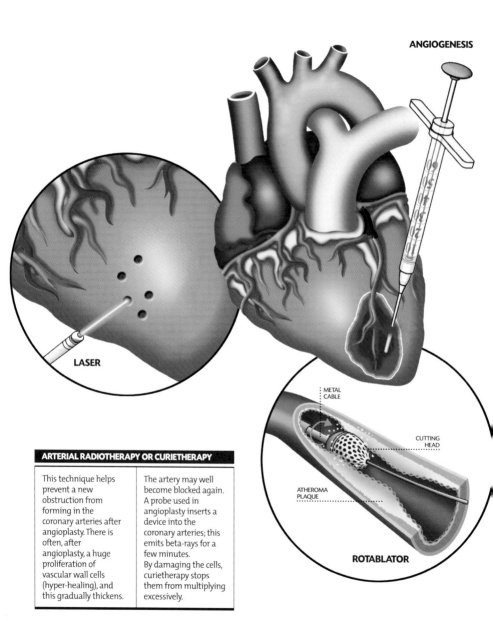

**ANGIOGENESIS**

**LASER**

**METAL CABLE**

**CUTTING HEAD**

**ATHEROMA PLAQUE**

**ROTABLATOR**

## ARTERIAL RADIOTHERAPY OR CURIETHERAPY

This technique helps prevent a new obstruction from forming in the coronary arteries after angioplasty. There is often, after angioplasty, a huge proliferation of vascular wall cells (hyper-healing), and this gradually thickens.

The artery may well become blocked again. A probe used in angioplasty inserts a device into the coronary arteries; this emits beta-rays for a few minutes. By damaging the cells, curietherapy stops them from multiplying excessively.

# New treatments

## Angiogenesis, a treatment for the future

In the United States, 1,000 patients suffering from persistent cardiac insufficiency, despite repeated angioplasties and coronary bypasses, have already benefited from angiogenesis. A large number of them have seen their symptoms reduce appreciably.

## The rotablator

A probe guides a minute metal cutting head to the blocked part of the artery. The cutting head cuts through the atheroma plaque at a speed of 100,000 revolutions per minute.
The plaque is literally pulverised and debris is removed by the blood flow.

## Simpson's catheter

If the atheroma plaque is calcified and hardened, the balloon does not have the strength to crush it. A Simpson's catheter is therefore introduced via the femoral artery to try to cut away the atheroma. The plaque is destroyed by tiny pincers that gnaw into it gradually. The probe is moved to the blocked part of the artery and sucks up the debris.

Every branch of science is involved in improving the treatment of heart disease: chemistry, surgery, bio-mechanics, physics and genetics.

### The laser: physics helping the heart

This idea involves using a laser to cut a number of holes through the heart muscle. These tiny holes might fill up with blood and become new vessels. This is a new method that is still on the drawing board, but it may help to avoid coronary bypass surgery in the future. Results look encouraging, but there is a great deal more research to do.

### Angiogenesis: genetics helping the heart

This technique was created in 1998. Researchers showed that, if a gene coding for a vascular growth factor (VEGF), is injected directly into the coronary arteries, it can stimulate the creation of new vessels. Other genes can also be introduced into the heart muscle to stimulate the development of new blood vessels to supply the heart. The new vessels are so small that we cannot see them, even using the latest imaging techniques such as MRA (magnetic resonance angiography). Scintigraphy alone shows the resulting improvement in blood supply to the heart.

# What triggers a heart attack?

**S**tress, intense physical exercise or anger. A heart attack can occur as a result of a particular event. But, more often, there is no single triggering factor, though it is known that attacks happen more frequently early in the morning or afternoon.

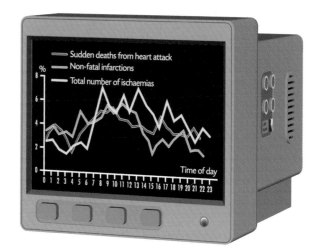

— Sudden deaths from heart attack
— Non-fatal infarctions
— Total number of ischaemias

Time of day

**FACTORS TRIGGERING AN INFARCTION**

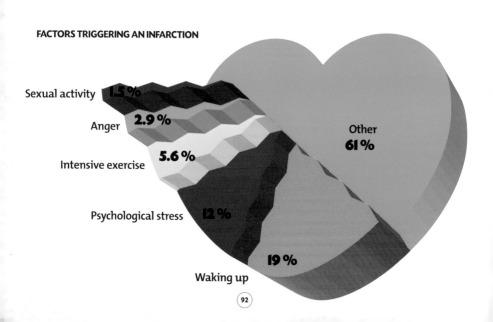

Sexual activity **1.5%**

Anger **2.9%**

Intensive exercise **5.6%**

Psychological stress **12%**

Waking up **19%**

Other **61%**

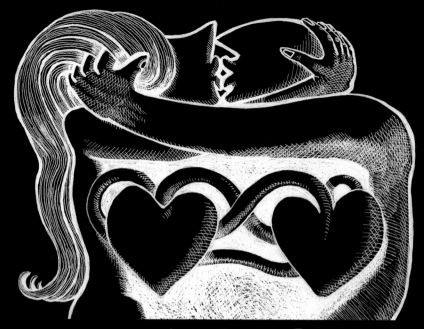

# FIND OUT

HOW CAN WE KEEP OUR HEARTS HEALTHY?
HOW TO CALCULATE YOUR RISK FACTORS. ADVICE FOR A HEALTHIER LIFE.
IF YOU DO HAVE A HEART ATTACK, HOW TO GET BACK TO A NORMAL LIFE.
TO HELP YOU FIND OUT MORE, THERE'S SOME ADVICE AND
USEFUL ADDRESSES AND WEBSITES IN THE FOLLOWING PAGES.

# *Doctor Zhivago*
# Boris Pasternak

**The fate of Yury Andreyevitch Zhivago is set against the turbulent backdrop of revolutionary Russia.**

He is orphaned at an early age and tries to build a life as a doctor. Exhausted after years of practising medicine, he finally succumbs to a heart attack after suffering an emotional shock.

'Yury sat on a single seat on the left, pressed against the window. He could see the left side of Nikita Street, the side of the Conservatoire. With the vague attention of a man thinking of something else, he watched the people walking and driving past on that side, missing no one. ...

Yury felt sick and faint. Overcoming his weakness, he got up and jerked the window straps up and down trying to open the window. But he could not move it.

People shouted to him that the window was blocked, it was nailed in position, but Yury, fighting off his faintness and seized by a sort of panic, neither understood the cries nor referred them to himself. He was still trying to open the window and again gave three sharp tugs at the strap – up, down and towards himself – when he suddenly felt a new and mortal pain, he understood that something had broken in him, he had done something irreparable and that this was the end. At this moment the tram started, but it had only gone a short way down Presnya Street when it stopped again.

By an inhuman effort of the will, Yury pushed through the solid crowd down the gangway, swaying and stumbling, and came out on the rear platform; people blocked his way and snapped at him. The fresh air seemed to revive him and he thought that perhaps not everything was lost, perhaps he was better.

He began to squeeze his way through the crush on the rear platform, provoking more snarls, curses and kicks. He paid no attention to them, tore himself free of the crowd, climbed down from the stationary tram into the roadway, took a step, another, a third, fell down on the cobbles and did not get up again.

There arose a hubbub of talk, arguments, advice. Several people got off the tram and surrounded him. They soon ascertained that he was no longer breathing: his heart had stopped. The group round the body was joined by others who stepped off the pavements, some relieved and others disappointed that the dead man had not been run over and that his death had nothing to do with the tram. ... '

© Collins Harvill, 1998

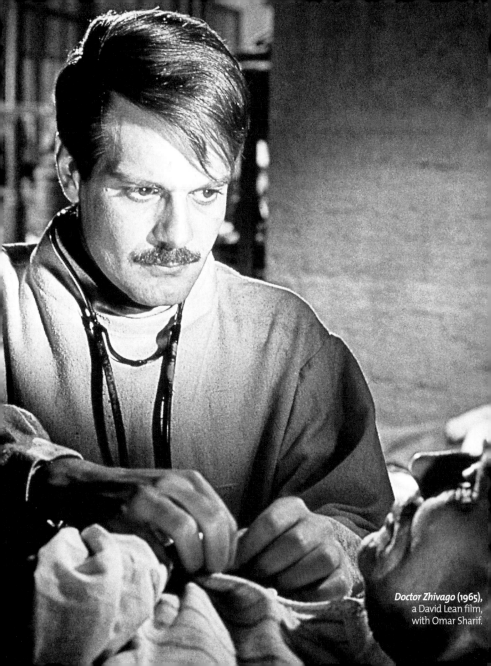

*Doctor Zhivago* (1965), a David Lean film, with Omar Sharif.

# Follow your heart ...

**To his heart's content**

**The heart is not only seen as the seat of the emotions; it is also at the heart of colloquial language and a source of inspiration for poets, who apply themselves wholeheartedly to the task ...**

**Learn by heart**

*My heart is like a singing bird*
*Whose nest is in a watered shoot;*
*My heart is like an apple-tree*
*Whose boughs are bent with thickset fruit;*
*My heart is like a rainbow shell*
*That paddles in a halcyon sea;*
*My heart is gladder than all these*
*Because my love is come to me.*

Christina Rossetti (*A Birthday*)

**His heart's in the right place**

**I've lost heart**

**It pulls at your heartstrings**

**Heartless**

**He wears his heart on his sleeve**

**Don't take it to heart**

**In my heart of hearts**

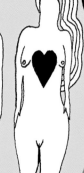
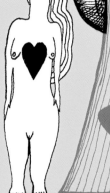
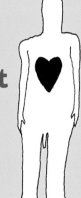

I lost my heart

It was heartening

# Take heart!

Pure in heart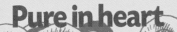

My heart was in my mouth

A heart of gold

A cry from the heart

Light-hearted

From the bottom of my heart

My heart's desire

To go straight to the heart of the matter

# A change of heart

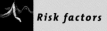
# Unavoidable risks

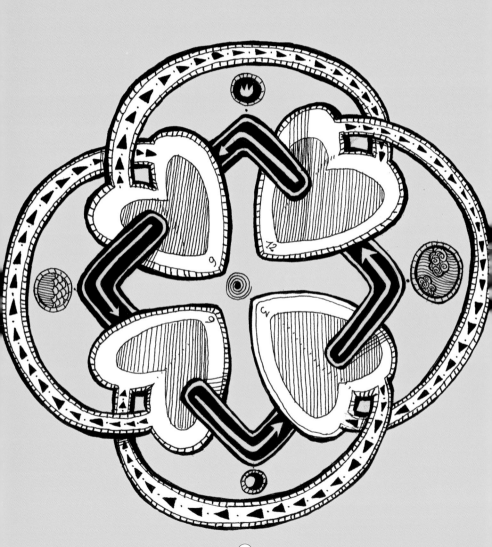

## Age

With every heartbeat, blood is pumped forcibly into the arteries.

As the years go by, the vessels put under this pressure start to harden and thicken, and deposits of fat and calcium may accumulate. This is why heart attacks occur more frequently in older people, especially over the age of 55. However, an attack is not inevitable. The risk can be limited by a healthy lifestyle.

## Sex

Women have some protection against heart attacks up to the menopause, thanks to oestrogens, which maintain the flexibility and elasticity of the vessels and thus restrict the formation of plaques of atherosclerosis. Oestrogens also have a beneficial effect on the liver, which secretes more good cholesterol or HDL, the role of which is to remove bad cholesterol or LDL from our blood. Therefore, the heart attack risk for a non-menopausal woman is five times lower than for a man of the same age. Hormone replacement therapy, based on oestrogens and progesterone and taken after the menopause, appears to protect women against heart disease in later years. Women generally experience their first heart attack at a more advanced age than men – by an average of ten years. Their greater age can mean that their bodies are less able to withstand a heart attack.

For these reasons, fatal heart attacks at all ages occur more frequently in women. In the first year after a heart attack, the death rate for women is 42 per cent, against only 24 per cent in men. But these figures only have a relative value: they do not take account of the advanced age of women, and therefore their greater fragility, when suffering their first heart attack.

## Heredity

Heredity plays a significant part in whether or not you are susceptible to heart disease. Anyone with close family members (parents, grandparents, siblings) who are suffering from angina pectoris or have had a heart attack at a young age (under 60 years) is classified as having a higher risk of suffering from heart disease themselves. Strokes are also more likely.

More than half of those affected by heart disease have close relatives who have suffered the same disease. The risk is even greater if the relative developed the disease before the age of 60.

# Smoking-related heart risks

**We need to do all we can to control those risks over which we can have some influence. It's up to us to keep our hearts as healthy as possible.**

## Tobacco: enemy no. 1

Smoking is one of the prime causes of death throughout the modern world. Directly or indirectly, it causes heart attacks, strokes, throat and lung cancers, respiratory problems such as emphysema and chronic bronchitis, and peripheral vascular insufficiency which leads to gangrene.

Smoking is currently recognised as one of the leading cardiovascular risk factors; it increases the risk of heart attack or angina pectoris by 70 per cent. When smoking, carbon dioxide replaces oxygen in red blood cells, so lowering the amount of oxygen the heart receives. Smoking is thought also to encourage premature ageing of the arteries and the formation of atherosclerotic areas.

## Nicotine

This is the cause of tobacco poisoning and of tobacco dependency. All of its effects are harmful. Smoking increases the heart rate and therefore the heart's daily workload. It has a vasoconstrictive effect, ie it reduces the diameter of the arteries, thus allowing less blood, and therefore less oxygen, to pass through.

Nicotine also helps increase the blood's viscosity, or thickness, thus making it easier for clots to form.

Lastly, it reduces the amount of good cholesterol or HDL and increases the amount of bad cholesterol or LDL, which collects on the vascular walls, encouraging atherosclerosis.

## How many cigarettes can I smoke?

The risk of a heart attack increases with the number of cigarettes smoked and the number of years spent smoking. On the other hand, pipe or cigar smokers, who do not inhale the smoke, run a lesser but nevertheless tangible risk.

It would appear that, after many years of abstinence, former smokers may return to a heart attack risk level equivalent to that of someone who has never smoked. However, we should temper our enthusiasm, as these statistics are global and do not enable us to predict the risk on an individual level.

## Women: the recent victims of smoking

Cigarettes are the most highly advertised product in the world. A large part of this advertising is aimed at women and, since 1987, lung cancer has been killing more women than breast cancer.

## Stop smoking!

### Be decisive

Try deciding in advance the day on which you're going to stop smoking. Choosing an anniversary or significant date of some sort is a good idea. But you've got to stick to it! Let your friends, family and work colleagues know of your decision and of the date. That will give you a little extra impetus to stick at it.

### Give yourself an incentive

Boost your willpower by making a list of the reasons you want to give up smoking. You can look at this list whenever the craving for a cigarette becomes strong. Work out how much money you will save by not smoking, and promise yourself a treat with this saved money.

### Be prepared

You've had a cigarette in your mouth several times a day for a long time, so you need to find some kind of substitute: try chewing gum, nibble on a carrot or drink lots of water. Identify those moments in the day when you normally smoke most, for example watching the TV or sitting at the computer, and take your psychological 'props' with you so that they'll be there at the crucial moment! Don't sit around doing nothing; take up a sport and you won't feel such a strong need to smoke. Don't stay at home; try to get out as much as possible. Lastly, try to organise a few outings with friends who don't smoke.

### Bridge the gap

Nicotine is a genuine drug, and smoking creates a dependency that makes it hard to give up tobacco. Nicotine withdrawal reveals itself in the form of anxiety, irritability, insomnia, concentration problems and, of course, an overwhelming desire to smoke. Nicotine patches or chewing gum can work very effectively to bridge this gap. They are usually prescribed for ten to twelve weeks and can thus lead to a gradual reduction in the daily supply of nicotine to the body. Talk to your doctor before you start to use them. There can sometimes be contra-indications for people suffering from severe heart disease.

Above all, don't smoke while you're using nicotine patches or chewing gum! Some antidepressants have recently been found to reduce the symptoms of nicotine shortage. Talk to your doctor about them.

# High blood pressure: a stealthy killer

## The new World Health Organization (WHO) classification

Hypertension or high blood pressure is defined by figures higher than 140/90 mm Hg. The higher figure, or systolic pressure, is measured during heart contraction, when blood is forcibly pumped through the body. It thus represents the highest pressure that our vessels have to withstand during each heartbeat. The lower figure (eg 90 mm of mercury – a column of mercury is still used in a blood pressure machine, or sphygmomanometer, to measure the body's blood pressure), or diastolic pressure, is measured when the heart is relaxed. It represents the lowest pressure that our vessels have to withstand, even at rest. These two figures are very important; you can have high systolic blood pressure, where only the maximum figure is high, high diastolic blood pressure, where only the minimum figure is high, which is often the case in older people, or you can have blood pressure affecting both figures. These three types of high blood pressure all contribute to the same problem: atherosclerosis, hardening of the arteries. In all cases, high blood pressure must be treated to reduce the likelihood of having a heart attack or stroke.

## Diagnosis

A single blood pressure measurement is not enough to make a diagnosis. In certain circumstances, it is perfectly normal for blood pressure to rise. In particular, so-called 'the white coat' phenomenon is well known, when blood pressure rises as soon as you arrive at the surgery due to anxiety over what the doctor will do or say. So, blood pressure must be measured several times and in the right conditions, ie sitting still, after a few moments' rest. Once you are over 40 years of age, it is recommended that you have your blood pressure checked every year. High blood pressure is classed as a disease, even though you may not feel any symptoms. There are plenty of effective treatments available, once it has been detected. Talk to your doctor about it.

Some studies have shown that normalisation of high blood pressure reduces strokes by 30 per cent, coronary thromboses by 35 per cent and cardiac insufficiency by 50 per cent.

## A silent disease

High blood pressure damages the arteries, causing them to harden and thicken. Although severe high blood pressure may cause headaches, shortness of breath, dizziness and disturbed vision, there are usually no symptoms. The disease often runs in families, and is more likely to develop in obese people, the elderly, or those with a sedentary lifestyle.

| THE NEW WHO CLASSIFICATION | | |
| --- | --- | --- |
| | MAXI<br>Systolic pressure<br>in mm of mercury | MINI<br>Diastolic pressure<br>in mm of mercury |
| **Optimum pressure** | < 120 | < 80 |
| **Upper limit of pressure** | > 130 | > 85 |
| **Slightly high blood pressure (1st degree)** | 140–160 | 90–100 |
| **Moderately high blood pressure (2nd degree)** | 160–180 | 100–110 |
| **Very high blood pressure (3rd degree)** | > 180 | > 110 |

## The consequences of high blood pressure

### On the heart
• Cardiac insufficiency: the heart grows larger in order to try to pump blood against the high pressures, until it is unable to push blood against the pressures, and actually becomes weaker
• Symptom: rapid breathlessness, especially when lying down.

• Infarction: death of heart cells due to blockage of the coronary arteries.
• Symptoms: serious chest pain, cold sweats.

### On the brain
• Brain haemorrhage: the pressure is too great for weakened blood vessels; they burst and bleed.
• Symptom: if small, there may be no symptoms. Larger bleeds may cause pain or symptoms of stroke like paralysis.
• Infarction: death of brain cells due to a blood clot in the cerebral arteries.
• Symptom: sudden paralysis.

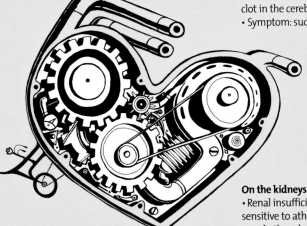

### On the kidneys
• Renal insufficiency: the kidneys are very sensitive to atherosclerosis. With poor blood supply, they shrink, then stop working.
• Symptoms: frequent urination, nausea and vomiting.

| WORK OUT YOUR OVERALL CARDIOVASCULAR RISK | | | |
|---|---|---|---|
| | DEGREE OF HIGH BLOOD PRESSURE | | |
| RISK | 1ST DEGREE | 2ND DEGREE | 3RD DEGREE |
| No factors | Slight risk | Average risk | High risk |
| 2 factors | Average risk | Average risk | Very high risk |
| 3 factors | High risk | High risk | Very high risk |
| Cardio-vascular disease | Very high risk | Very high risk | Very high risk |

### Don't forget the other risk factors
Age, sex, heredity, high cholesterol, diabetes, smoking, obesity, and sedentary lifestyle – these don't just add to the risk; they multiply them!

# Do you know your cholesterol level?

**Cholesterol is a natural lipid (or fat) that is indispensable to the body. In order to circulate in the blood, cholesterol attaches itself to different proteins known as lipoproteins, two of which are HDLs and LDLs.**

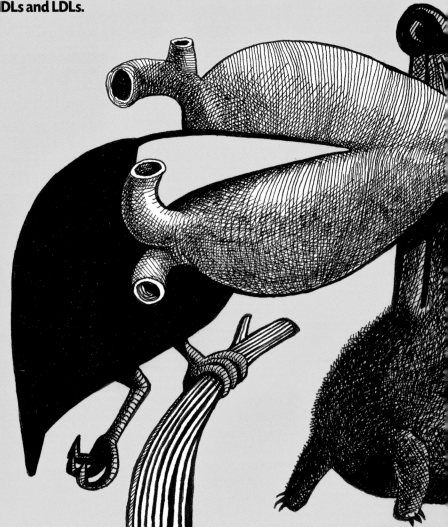

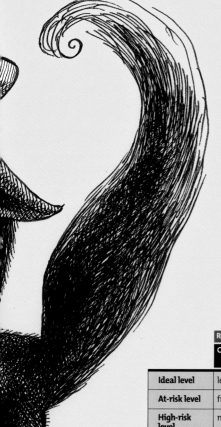

## HDLs, or good cholesterol

HDL proteins (high density lipoprotein) fix cholesterol and transport it to the liver, where it is eliminated or used up. HDLs are useful. They clean the blood and the vessels of excess cholesterol. So, good cholesterol protects humans against risks of heart disease.

## LDLs, or bad cholesterol

LDL proteins (low density lipoprotein) also fix cholesterol but, once they have done so, they attach themselves to the walls of blood vessels. Fatty deposits build up and partially block arteries.

The LDL level in the blood is therefore a good indicator of cardiovascular risk. The higher the level, the greater the risk of problems.

## Hypercholesterolaemia (high cholesterol levels)

A blood cholesterol level above 5 mmol/l is considered high.

This measurement should always be adjusted according to age as cholesterol rises with age.

## Checking for lipids

This consists of measuring amounts of total cholesterol, triglycerides and sometimes HDLs and LDLs on an empty stomach. An annual check-up is recommended if there is any cause for concern .

Hereditary forms of hypercholesterolaemia (high blood cholesterol levels) can be very serious. Children should be encouraged to follow a healthy diet from an early age.

| RECOMMENDED CHOLESTEROL LEVELS | | |
|---|---|---|
| | CHOLESTEROL | HDL | LDL |
| **Ideal level** | less than 2 g/l | 0.4 to 0.55 | less than 1.3 g/l |
| **At-risk level** | from 2 to 2.4 g/l | | from 1.3 to 1.6g/l |
| **High-risk level** | more than 2.4 g/l | less than 0.35 g/l | more than 1.6g/l |

# Diabetes multiplies the risk of heart disease four to seven times

**On an empty stomach, blood sugar level should be less than 7 mmol/l. If this level is above 7 mmol/l in two consecutive tests, doctors begin to suspect diabetes.**

### Two types of diabetes

Maturity onset diabetes, or Type 2 diabetes, affects two to three per cent of the overall population and up to 20 per cent of people aged over 80. The disease is often hereditary: up to 20 per cent of the members of a family may be afflicted. Known as the mature person's diabetes, it often starts after the age of 40 and, in 70 per cent of cases, is linked to obesity.

This form of diabetes is probably a result of reduced insulin-sensitivity in the tissues, especially the muscles. Insulin's function is to transfer sugar from the blood into the cells. It thus supplies the cells with their main source of energy and reduces blood sugar level. If insulin is unable to work effectively, blood sugar level increases, especially when high-energy-containing food is eaten.

The overworked pancreas becomes exhausted and can no longer make enough insulin. The progression of diabetes is usually contained by diet and weight loss. However, in some cases insulin production by the pancreas continues to fall and eventually drugs have to be prescribed to control blood sugar.

Insulin-dependent diabetes (Type 1 diabetes) is much more rare: fortunately it affects only 0.5 per cent of the population. It often affects several members of the same family, but its hereditary component is not well defined. This form of diabetes starts in infancy, adolescence and early adulthood. It is the result of a complete failure in the manufacture of insulin. It can, therefore, only be treated by daily insulin injections.

### Diabetes and atherosclerosis

Excess blood sugar damages the vascular wall, which loses its elasticity, thus attracting deposits of fat and calcium, as well as fibrous deposits inside the blood vessels. Blocked arteries can no longer supply blood to the organs.

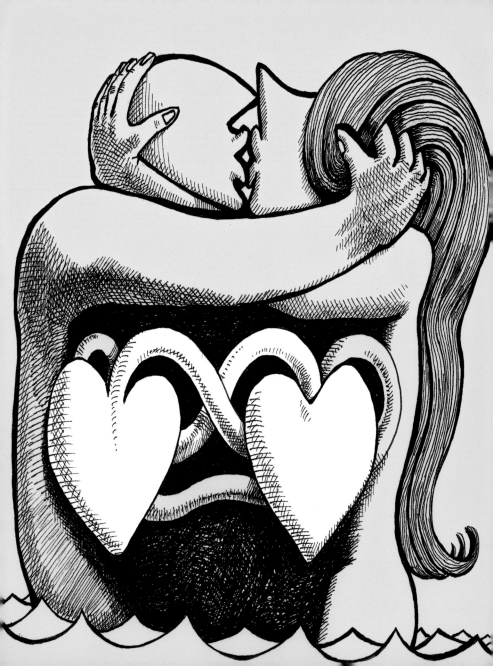

# Other risk factors

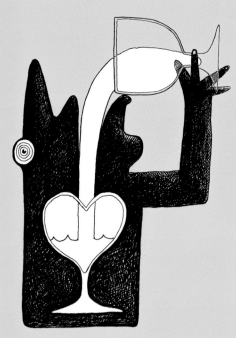

Stress, whether physical or emotional, suddenly increases the heart's workload. Catecholamines (stress proteins), which include adrenalin, make the heart beat faster than normal and raise blood pressure. As a result, the heart needs more oxygen and, if the coronary arteries are blocked, this demand cannot be met. Angina pectoris or a heart attack may follow.

**WATCH YOUR WEIGHT!**

*Obesity is defined as a weight that is 30 per cent higher than normal weight. It is often linked to a sedentary lifestyle, age-onset diabetes, high blood pressure and hypercholesterolaemia. In addition, it increases the level of bad cholesterol and decreases the level of good cholesterol. In contrast, weight loss often helps to 'cure' high blood pressure, diabetes and hypercholesterolaemia. It also makes taking exercise easier. Normal weight can only benefit the heart.*

### Alcohol: for better or for worse

The rate of death from heart disease fluctuates very much in line with the amount of fat in the diet throughout the world. The exception to this is France where, despite the heaviness of French cuisine with all its sauces, the French suffer less from heart disease. Several studies have shown that moderate red wine consumption (one glass a day) is at the root of this paradox, but equally it should be said that too much alcohol causes chronic heart muscle disease, leading to cardiac insufficiency – and many other problems beyond the heart!

### IDEAL WEIGHT FOR YOUR HEIGHT AND SEX

| HEIGHT | MEN | WOMEN |
|---|---|---|
| 5 ft/1.50 m | 110 lb/50 kg | 110 lb/50 kg |
| 5 ft 2 in/1.55 m | 118 lb/54 kg | 115 lb/52.5 kg |
| 5 ft 3 in/1.60 m | 127 lb/57.5 kg | 121 lb/55 kg |
| 5 ft 5 in/1.65 m | 134 lb/61.5 kg | 127 lb/57.5 kg |
| 5 ft 7 in/1.70 m | 144 lb/65 kg | 132 lb/60 kg |
| 5 ft 9 in/1.75 m | 152 lb/69 kg | 137 lb/62.5 kg |
| 5 ft 11 in/1.80 m | 159 lb/72.5 kg | 142 lb/65 kg |
| 6 ft 1 in/1.85 m | 168 lb/76.5 kg | 149 lb/67.5 kg |
| 6 ft 3 in/1.90 m | 176 lb/80 kg | 154 lb/70 kg |
| 6 ft 3 in/1.90 m | 176 lb/80 kg | 154 lb/70 kg |

# New risks for the heart: bacteria and proteins

## Microbes that attack our arteries

Researchers have recently detected a number of micro-organisms that may be responsible for heart diseases. However, the results of current studies remain as yet unconfirmed.

### Stomach ulcer bacteria

Infection with *Helicobacter pylori* bacteria could create inflammation in the coronary arteries and lead to atherosclerosis. The bacterium has been found in 62 per cent of patients suffering from coronary artery disease, compared with 40 per cent in people not suffering from the disease.
Antibiotic treatment may be effective, but concrete evidence has yet to be collected.

## Proteins that attack the heart

Fibrinogen and lipoprotein A are both natural proteins. High levels of either are usually hereditary. Amongst other things they encourage the formation of blood clots responsible for heart attacks. Lipoprotein A also encourages the formation of atheroma plaques. These are two separate heart risk factors.

### Homocysteine

When its level in the blood is too high, this natural amino acid damages the vascular walls. A study of 14,000 doctors, carried out at Harvard in 1992, showed that homocysteine increases the risk of heart attack by three times.
An increase in the level of homocysteine is often hereditary: one person in eight carries a gene that slows down metabolism, increasing the level of homocysteine in the blood.

# Your place in society

One of the more disturbing results to emerge from an analysis of premature deaths by coronary heart disease is that manual workers are significantly more at risk than non-manual workers, sometimes by as much as 100 per cent. This statistical imbalance cannot, of course, be attributed to any one factor: the lifestyle associated with a low income and a lower level of education is to blame. Manual workers and their children are less likely to eat the recommended daily levels of fruit and vegetables, and more likely to eat fatty foods. They are also more likely to smoke: 34 per cent are smokers compared with 21 per cent of non-manual workers. Obesity and the absence of a supportive social network, another factor that has been linked to heart disease, are also more prevalent among manual workers.

## Where you live

More people suffer heart disease in northern Britain and Northern Ireland than in Wales and the south of England. Ethnic south Asians living in the UK are also more likely to suffer than the rest of the population. The UK as a whole has a very high rate of heart disease compared with other countries, though higher rates are recorded in some eastern European countries.

# Physical activity: advantages for the heart

**Physical activity benefits the heart, reducing blood pressure and releasing pent-up energy. This may be especially beneficial for what are known as 'Type A' personalities. According to research, Type A individuals have a strong competitive urge. They are highly productive and put a lot into their work, often just for the pleasure of winning. They are stimulated by deadlines. Headstrong, sharp, often impatient and even bad-tempered, they can be quite aggressive. Unfortunately modern industrial society tends to encourage this sort of behaviour, which may be harmful to health.**

## Your heart needs exercise

High cholesterol, smoking and high blood pressure are certainly high risk factors for the heart. But we must not forget that lack of exercise is also dangerous for our health and especially for the heart.

## The benefits of exercise

Taking exercise improves blood circulation, including blood supply to the heart, thereby reducing the risk of heart attack.

Sport prevents or reduces high blood pressure, reduces hyperglycaemia and increases the level of HDLs, or good cholesterol, in the blood. In addition, physical activity helps control and limit weight gain. Lastly, smokers smoke much less when they take exercise.

Having a regular physical activity increases energy, reduces stress and strengthens the bones. Physical activity also gives a feeling of well-being by increasing production of endorphins, types of natural morphine synthesised in the body.

## Sport for all

Sport is essential for everybody, including the elderly. It can even prevent certain chronic illnesses associated with old age. Practising a sport also helps reduce the period of convalescence after illness and encourages physical independence.

## What sort of exercise should I do?

Aerobic exercises are best for the heart and lungs. These include fast walking (two steps per second), running, swimming, cycling, ice-skating, roller-skating or cross-country skiing. These sports exercise the leg and arm muscles and accelerate our heart rhythm effectively by increasing heart output.

Bodybuilding and other exercises using weights and barbells are known as isometric exercises. Excessive practice is not recommended for the heart as it can cause sudden increases in blood pressure, accelerate heart rate and workload abruptly and for only a short period, with the result that the heart does not have time to adjust.

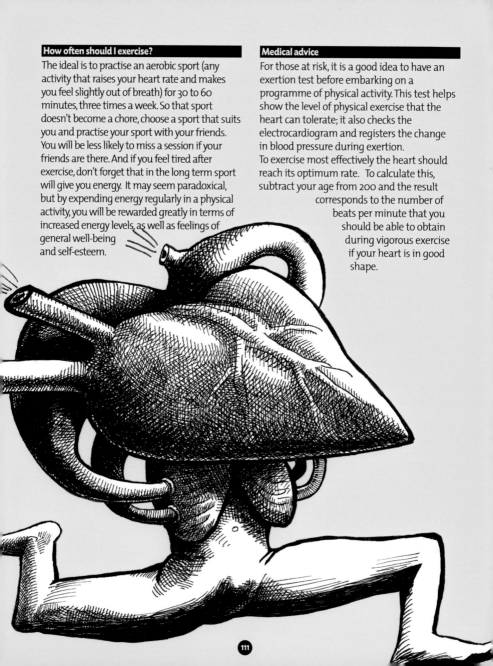

## How often should I exercise?

The ideal is to practise an aerobic sport (any activity that raises your heart rate and makes you feel slightly out of breath) for 30 to 60 minutes, three times a week. So that sport doesn't become a chore, choose a sport that suits you and practise your sport with your friends. You will be less likely to miss a session if your friends are there. And if you feel tired after exercise, don't forget that in the long term sport will give you energy. It may seem paradoxical, but by expending energy regularly in a physical activity, you will be rewarded greatly in terms of increased energy levels, as well as feelings of general well-being and self-esteem.

## Medical advice

For those at risk, it is a good idea to have an exertion test before embarking on a programme of physical activity. This test helps show the level of physical exercise that the heart can tolerate; it also checks the electrocardiogram and registers the change in blood pressure during exertion.

To exercise most effectively the heart should reach its optimum rate. To calculate this, subtract your age from 200 and the result corresponds to the number of beats per minute that you should be able to obtain during vigorous exercise if your heart is in good shape.

# The importance of diet

**The people of Crete are great consumers of olive oil, fish, vegetables, fruit and garlic, but they eat very few dairy products and cakes, and very little red meat. They live longer than anyone else in Europe and have the lowest level of cardiovascular disease. According to some research, the consumption of half a clove of garlic or three apples a day significantly reduces total cholesterol level.**

## The advantages and disadvantages of lipids

Most fats, or lipids, are vital to a balanced diet. But eating too much saturated fat or cholesterol-rich food increases the level of bad cholesterol (LDL), which is deposited on the artery walls and helps cause atherosclerosis. The body manufactures a sufficient amount of these fats, so we only need to ingest them in very small quantities. In contrast, unsaturated lipids and essential fatty acids increase good cholesterol (HDL), which clears plaques of fat out of our arteries. This is why certain foods are preferable to others. Olive oil is rich in mono-unsaturated fatty acids that reduce bad cholesterol. Fish is rich in Omega 3 fatty acids.

Omega 3 lowers the level of cholesterol and triglycerides (other lipids circulating in the blood) and prevents blood platelet stimulation and therefore blood clot formation. It also helps regulate high blood pressure.

## HOW TO REDUCE YOUR CHOLESTEROL LEVEL

| FOODS TO AVOID | HEALTHIER FOODS |
|---|---|
| • *Fried food: grill, bake or poach food instead.*<br>• *Processed food: crisps, cakes, puddings, etc.*<br>• *Red meat (beef, pork, lamb).*<br>• *Offal and cooked meats; remove fat from meat and skin from poultry.*<br>• *Egg yolks, which are high in cholesterol.*<br>• *Butter.* | • *Chicken, turkey, fish.*<br>• *Fibre-rich foods, such as vegetables (lentils, beans), cereals, fruit (also rich in vitamins).*<br>• *Goose fat, olive oil and sunflower oil rather than tropical oils (coca, palm).*<br>• *Skimmed dairy products (milk, cheese).* |

## Fruit, vegetables and dietary fibre

Fruit and vegetables are rich in vitamins and minerals, and low in calories and fats. They help protect us from heart attacks and also from some cancers (especially of the colon). Dietary fibre is that part of a plant that we cannot digest; it may be soluble or insoluble. Soluble fibre helps us to reduce our cholesterol level. It is found in cereals, beans, peas, lentils, citrus fruit (lemons, oranges), strawberries and apples.
Insoluble fibre does not alter our cholesterol level, but it aids digestion. It is found in wholemeal bread, cereals, carrots, Brussels sprouts, cauliflower, beetroot, prunes and the skins of apples.

## Antioxidants

Bad cholesterol, or LDL, damages our arteries in a variety of ways, including oxidation reactions. Oxidation makes atheroma plaques more liquid and unstable. With this in mind, a number of research projects in recent years have focused on antioxidant molecules that might help reduce the risk of heart attacks and strokes. It appears currently that vitamin E might be most likely to combat oxidation. Vitamin E is found in dried fruit, cereals and green vegetables.

Vitamin C, selenium, carotene and gingko biloba extracts may also be useful in the fight against atherosclerosis by preventing oxidisation. Vitamin C is found in raw fruit and vegetables (cooking destroys it). Carotene is found in carrots, melons and broccoli. Selenium is a mineral most often found in seafood products.

## Salt

Salt, or sodium chloride (NaCl), is the most abundant mineral compound circulating in the blood. It helps retain water in the body and avoid dehydration. Most of us do not need to follow a low-salt diet. We can prevent excess by simply not adding more salt to our food. But people suffering from high blood pressure or cardiac insufficiency may benefit from reducing their salt intake, as increased salt pushes blood pressure higher and puts a greater strain on the heart.

## Potassium and magnesium are vital in helping the heart beat regularly

A low level of potassium or magnesium may cause serious heart rhythm disorders. Diuretics are often prescribed in cases of high blood pressure or cardiac insufficiency. By increasing urine secretion, they lead to a considerable loss of these two minerals in the urine. Potassium and/or magnesium tablets are therefore sometimes given to prevent a possible imbalance. Also, diarrhoea and vomiting may seriously reduce your potassium level.

# Work out your heart attack risk

**This test will help you establish your cardiovascular profile. It takes into account those risks over which you have no control (heredity, sex, age) and those that you can do something about (smoking, cholesterol, weight, high blood pressure).**

## Sex

| | |
|---|---|
| Woman under 40 | 1 point |
| Woman aged 40 to 50 | 2 points |
| Woman over 50 | 3 points |
| Man | 5 points |
| Well built man | 6 points |
| Bald, well built man | 7 points |

## Age

| | |
|---|---|
| 10 to 20 years | 1 point |
| 21 to 30 | 2 points |
| 31 to 40 | 3 points |
| 41 to 50 | 4 points |
| 51 to 60 | 6 points |
| 61 upwards | 8 points |

## Blood pressure (systolic values)

| | |
|---|---|
| 100 | 1 point |
| 120 | 2 points |
| 140 | 3 points |
| 160 | 4 points |
| 180 | 6 points |
| 200 and upwards | 8 points |

## Weight*

| | |
|---|---|
| Less than 2.5 kg/5 lbs 7 oz above normal weight | 0 points |
| Up to 2.5 kg/5 lbs 7 oz above normal weight | 1 point |
| 3 to 10 kg/6 to 22 lbs above normal weight | 2 points |
| 10 to 16 kg/22 to 35 lbs above normal weight | 3 points |
| 18 to 25 kg/35 to 55lbs above normal weight | 5 points |
| 25 to 32 kg/55 to 70 lbs above normal weight | 7 points |

* TO FIND OUT YOUR IDEAL WEIGHT, SEE TABLE ON P. 108.

# Cardiac heredity

| | |
|---|---|
| None | 1 point |
| One close relative who has suffered cardiovascular disease over the age of 60 | 2 points |
| Two close relatives who have suffered cardiovascular disease over the age of 60 | 3 points |
| One close relative who has suffered cardiovascular disease under the age of 60 | 4 points |
| Two close relatives who have suffered cardiovascular disease under the age of 60 | 6 points |
| Three close relatives who have suffered cardiovascular disease under the age of 60 | 7 points |

# Smoking

| | |
|---|---|
| Non-smoker | 0 points |
| Cigar and/or pipe | 1 point |
| 10 cigarettes a day | 2 points |
| 20 cigarettes a day | 4 points |
| 30 cigarettes a day | 6 points |
| 40 cigarettes or more a day | 10 points |

# Diet

| | |
|---|---|
| No butter, no oil, no eggs | 1 point |
| Grilled meat with vegetables, few eggs and very little fat | 2 points |
| Normal diet with eggs, but no fried food or sauces | 3 points |
| Normal diet with some fried food, sauces and fats | 4 points |
| Rich diet with sauces, fried food and cakes | 5 points |
| Diet contains large amounts of sauces, fried food and cakes | 7 points |

# Exercise

| | |
|---|---|
| Active work, intensive exercise | 1 point |
| Active work, moderate exercise | 2 points |
| Sedentary work, intensive exercise | 3 points |
| Sedentary work, moderate exercise | 5 points |
| Sedentary work, little exercise | 6 points |
| Total lack of exercise | 8 points |

**ADD UP YOUR POINTS**

*6 to 11 points: very low risk*
*12 to 17: low risk*
*18 to 24: a certain risk, but not too worrying*
*25 to 31: careful, you are at risk*
*32 to 40: you are at considerable risk*
*41 to 62: you are in the high-risk category. See a doctor.*

Source : French Cardiology Federation.

# Taking your life in hand after a heart attack

**It is vital to rehabilitate the heart after a heart attack. This is done initially under medical supervision, but after a few weeks, you must learn to take control of your day-to-day life again.**

## In hospital

In the absence of complications, the length of time spent in hospital after a heart attack is about a week. Usually, the patient spends the first two days in intensive care or in a coronary care unit with sensitive heart monitoring. He is then transferred to the cardiology or medical wards.

## Effective treatments

Anti-platelet drugs (such as aspirin), ACE inhibitors, beta-blockers and statins have proved effective in preventing recurrence of a heart attack, which is often fatal. Aspirin is usually prescribed in small doses, 75 to 160 mg/day; the normal adult dose for headaches is 300 to 900 mg, three times a day. This low dosage is perfectly effective and does not usually cause stomach problems. Aspirin at the same dosage level also prevents strokes. After angioplasty, it may be necessary to prescribe anti-platelet drugs more powerful than aspirin. Statins are major cholesterol-lowering agents. In addition to their exceptional preventive effects, they can also stabilise crumbling atheroma plaques, which might otherwise suddenly block the coronary arteries. As a result, they reduce the coronary death rate by around 30 per cent. Lastly, statins effectively prevent re-obstruction after angioplasty.

## Some advice before you return home

Learn to take your pulse.
Feel your pulse at the wrist and count the beats for 15 seconds. Multiply the result by four. Your heart should beat regularly between 50 and 100 times a minute. Call your doctor if you have palpitations, or if your heart is beating irregularly or too fast.

## Recognise your symptoms

Call your doctor if you are breathless or if you have leg swelling, chest pain, dizziness, cold sweats, nausea or vomiting.

## Take precautions

Any physical activity requires energy and increases the heart's workload. For a few weeks after a heart attack, try not to go upstairs too quickly, lift weights or do anything physical after a meal. Sexual activity also involves a fairly high energy output; it is therefore better to abstain for a month after a heart attack.

## How to cope with a heart attack

It is usual to feel depressed and morally and physically weakened after a heart attack. The attack came suddenly and has completely changed your life, so you will need to change some of your habits. You must stop smoking, follow a light, balanced diet, do some sport, check your blood pressure regularly, and take care to keep your cholesterol level within limits.
Discuss your concerns with your doctor, with people at the rehabilitation centre, or your family.

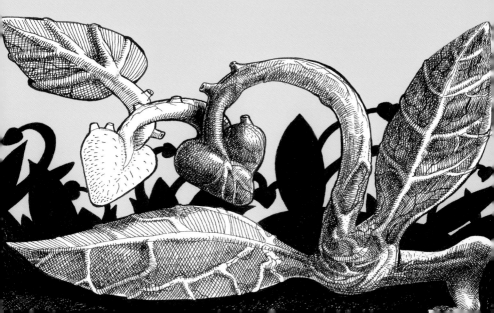

# Heart FAQs:
# some frequently asked questions

### I lead a healthy life; why have I had a heart attack?

Excess fat, smoking and alcohol do influence the sudden occurrence of a heart attack, but they are not the only risk factors. Stress is just as important, it puts us 'under pressure' and makes the heart work too hard. Lastly, faced with disease, we are all unequal; heredity and age count for or against us.

### I have a heart condition; can I take the Pill?

You can take the pill if your blood pressure and triglyceride (a fat whose level in the blood is measured) counts allow you to. You are strongly advised not to smoke if you choose this form of contraception. If you have had a heart attack, or are at high risk, you will be offered other forms of contraception. If your heart condition is worrying you, consult a doctor.

### I have a heart condition; can I continue to drive my car?

Yes. Once you have stabilised, you can gradually return to normal life with all the exertions that that entails, such as driving your car or going upstairs.

While you can drive your car quite soon after leaving hospital, lorry drivers are advised not to drive their lorries for several weeks, especially if they are involved in the loading and unloading of the lorry.

### I have a heart condition; can I be vaccinated?

Yes.

### I have a heart condition; can I continue to give blood?

The transfusion centre will carry out a preliminary investigation, especially if you are taking medication. If you have had a heart attack, you cannot normally give blood for at least a year. The same applies if you suffer from cardiac insufficiency or high blood pressure during certain treatments.

### Are there any products that are toxic to someone with a heart condition?

Volatile toxic products, for example lighter fuel, some adhesives containing acetone or powerful solvents may cause irritation leading to palpitations. You should avoid exposure to such products, whether you have a heart condition or not.

### I have diabetes; do I risk having a heart condition?

You have diabetes, so your risk is increased. If you are overweight, you should try first of all to lose weight; this will help you bring your diabetes under control. Diabetes contributes to damage of the artery walls and formation of atherosclerosis of the coronary arteries and so increases the risk of heart disease. You must be careful to keep your diabetes firmly under control.

### Is it dangerous for me to go out in the sun?

The sun is not dangerous in small doses. On the other hand, it is not good to spend several hours exposed to the midday sun. Heat causes dilation of the tiny blood vessels in the skin, heavy perspiration and an increase in the heart's workload and oxygen consumption.

So, spend only a short time in the sun. This precaution is not only valuable for the heart, but is important for protection against skin cancer, as well as premature ageing of the skin.

### Can I play sport after a heart attack?
Yes, once you have got back into your normal routine and an exertion test carried out at least a month after the heart attack shows what you are capable of. Sport should be practised regularly, but avoid sports that are too violent or that require sudden exertion (tennis, football, rugby) and, as a general rule, avoid competition. Try walking, cycling or swimming instead.

### Can I have sexual relations?
A return to normal physical activity means that you can return to regular sexual relations. However, after a heart attack, you should wait for around four weeks before having sexual relations.

### I have a heart condition; can I travel by air?
As long as the heart condition is under control, there is no reason why you should not travel by air.

### Should I take precautions as far as dental care is concerned?
Discuss this with your doctor and dentist. It all depends on the type of disease you have suffered. If you have heart valve disease, you must have antibiotic treatment before any dental extraction. If you are taking oral anticoagulants, you should stop the treatment about two days before you are to have dental treatment.
If this anticoagulant treatment is absolutely necessary, your doctor will prescribe an equivalent product that is administered subcutaneously (under the skin).

### Is it dangerous to sleep on your left side?
Whether you sleep on your left side, your right side or on your back, the heart's workload does not change. It may just happen that, if you are lying on your left side, you will hear the sound of your heartbeat transmitted by the mattress or the arm that you are lying on and so you become more conscious of it.

### Can I continue to have a sauna after heart disease?
It would be better not to, as any sudden change in temperature leads to a considerable increase in the heart's workload. But if you don't stay in for too long, and you have waited for a reasonable time after the heart attack, there is no particular reason why you should not have a sauna.

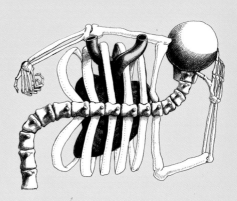

# Finding out

**BRITISH HEART
FOUNDATION**
14 Fitzhardinge Street
London W1H 4DH
Tel: 020 7935 0185
Fax: 020 7486 5820
www.bhf.org.uk

**BRITISH CARDIAC
SOCIETY**
9 Fitzroy Square
London W1P 5AH
Tel: 020 7383 3887
Fax: 020 7388 0903
E-mail:
enquiries@bcs.com
www.bcs.com

**CORONARY
PREVENTION GROUP**
The London School of
Hygiene
2 Taviton Street
London WC1H 0BT
Tel: 020 7636 8636

**NATIONAL HEART
RESEARCH FUND**
Concord House
Park Lane
Leeds LS3 1EQ
Tel: 0113 234 7474
Fax: 0113 297 6208
www.heartresearch.org.
uk

**BRISTOL HEART
INSTITUTE**
Level 7
Bristol Royal Infirmary
Upper Maudlin Street
Bristol BS2 8HW
Tel: 0117 928 3582
Fax: 0117 928 3581

**NHS DIRECT**
Tel: 0845 4647
www.nhsdirect.nhs.uk
*A nurse-staffed helpline for
any medical/health queries*

**UNIVERSITY OF OTTAWA
HEART INSTITUTE**
40 Ruskin Street
Ottawa, ON
K1Y 4W7
Canada
Tel: 001 613 761 5000
Fax: 001 613 761 5323
webmaster@ottawa
heart.ca
www.ottawaheart.ca

**AMERICAN HEART
ASSOCIATION**
National Center
7272 Greenville Avenue
Dallas, Texas 75231
USA

**TEXAS HEART
INSTITUTE**
1101 Bates Avenue
Houston
Texas 77030
USA
Tel: 001 713 791 4011
his@heart.thi.tmc.edu

**LINDA AND JACK GILL
HEART INSTITUTE**
University of Kentucky
Rose Street
Lexington KY 40536
USA
Tel: 001 859 257 9000
www.mc.uky.edu/ghi/

# Internet

**NATIONAL HEART
SUPPORT ASSOCIATION
– HEARTLINK**
www.heartlink.org.uk
*Support group*

**THE RESUSCITATION
COUNCIL**
www.resus.org.uk
*Provides education and
reference materials to
healthcare professionals
and the general public in
the most effective methods
of resuscitation.*

**THE HEALTH EDUCATION
AUTHORITY**
www.hea.org.uk

**THE DEPARTMENT OF
HEALTH HOME PAGE**
www.open.gov.uk/doh/
dhhome.html

**HEARTPOINT**
www.heartpoint.com
*Heartpoint was created by
medical professionals to
provide patients with a
source of credible information about heart disease.*

**CHEST, HEART AND
STROKE SCOTLAND**
65 North Castle Street
Edinburgh EH2 3LT
Tel: 0131 225 6963
Fax: 0131 220 6313
admin@chss.org.uk
www.chss.org.uk

**EUROPEAN HEART
NETWORK**
www.ehnheart.org

**EUROPEAN SOCIETY
OF CARDIOLOGY**
The European Heart
House
2035 Rte des Colles
B.P. 179, Les Templiers
FR-06903 Sophia
Antipolis
France
Tel: 00 33 4 92 94 76 00
Fax: 00 33 4 92 94 76 01
webmaster@escardio.org
www.escardio.org

**GLOBAL CARDIOLOGY
NETWORK**
www.globalcardiology.
org

**WORLD HEART
FEDERATION**
34 rue de l'Athénée
CH-1206 Geneva
Switzerland
Tel: 00 41 22 347 67 55
Fax: 00 41 22 347 10 28
www.worldheart.org

**WORLD HEART DAY**
www.worldheart.com

www.surgerydoor.co.uk
*Packed with information
and linked to the NHS*

www.netdoctor.co.uk

# Patient associations

**BRITISH CARDIAC
PATIENTS ASSOCIATION**
Unit 5D
2 Station Road
Swavesey
Cambridge CB4 5QJ
Tel: (helpline) 01223
846845 or 01223 247431
Tel./fax (administration)
01954 202022

# Further reading

Dr Graham Jackson, *Heart Health at your Fingertips*. Clan Publishing

Christopher Davidson, *Family Doctor Guide to Coronary Heart Disease* . Dorling Kindersley, 2000

Craig Donellan, ed. *Heart Disease* Issues Vol 48, Indpendence Educational Publishers, Cambridge, 2000

Tom Smith, *Heart Attacks: Prevent and Survive*, Sheldon Press, 1990

Eric Jager, *The Book of the Heart*, University of Chicago Press, 2000
Follows the history and psychology of emotion, concentrating on the concept of the heart, especially in the Middle Ages.

Milad Doveihi, *A Perverse History of the Human Heart*, Harvard University Press, 1998
The heart through custom, legend, religion and literature from ancient to modern times.

Stephen Westaby et al, *Landmarks in Cardiac Surgery*, Isis Medical, 1997

Stephen Klaidman, *Saving the Heart*, OUP (US) , 2000
The battle to conquer coronary heart disease.

*American College of Physicians Healthy Heart Cookbook*, Dorling Kindersley, 2000

Wilson S. Colucci (Ed.), *Atlas of Heart Failure: Cardiac Function & Dysfunction*, Sheridan House, 1999

Sally Edwards, *The Heart Rate Monitor Guidebook to Heart Zone Training*, Access Publishers Network, 1999
How to improve your health with the aid of a heart monitor.

Michio Kushi, Alex Jack, *Diet for a Strong Heart: Michio Kushi's Macrobiotic Dietary Guidelines for the Prevention of High Blood Pressure, Heart Attack, and Stroke*, St. Martin's Press, 1987

Marianne J. Legato, Carol Colman, *The Female Heart: The Truth About Women and Heart Disease,* HarperCollins, 2000

Candace McCarthy, Stobie Piel, Laurel Collins, *Affairs of the Heart*, Zebra Books, 1999
Three stories centred around St. Valentine's Day.

Thomas Moore (Ed.), *The Education of the Heart*, Hodder and Stoughton, 1998
A study of emotional intelligence in a technology-driven world.

M. Sara Rosenthal, *50 Ways Women Can Prevent Heart Disease*, Lowell House, 2000

Marc A. Silver, *Success With Heart Failure: Help and Hope for Those With Congestive Heart Failure*, Insight Books, 1998

Texas Heart Institute, Houston, USA, *Texas Heart Institute Heart Owner's Handbook*, John Wiley and Sons, 1996
How to live a longer and healthier life by looking after your heart.

Michael C. White, *The Blind Side of the Heart*, Cliff Street Books, 2001
A story about the enigma of the human heart and the layers of truth it is capable of hiding.'

Redford Williams, Virginia Williams, *Anger Kills: Seventeen Strategies for Controlling the Hostility That Can Harm Your Health*, HarperCollins, 1994

## *The heart versus the mind*

An age-old struggle, as this somewhat unpolitically correct quotation from Lord Chesterfield in his *Letters* of 1748 proves:
'The heart has such an influence over the understanding, that it is worth while to engage it in our interest. It is the whole of women, who are guided by nothing else: and it has so much to say, even with men, and the ablest of men too, that it commonly triumphs in every struggle with the understanding.'

## A

**ANEURYSM**

*Abnormal dilation of part of the vascular system (eg heart, artery). A heart aneurysm is a dilation of the heart cavity, which occurs in the weeks following an infarction. The consequences can be very serious.*

**ANGINA PECTORIS**

*Symptom of lack of oxygen to the heart; chest pain, often spreading to the arms, neck, jaw and back, usually on exertion.*

**ANGIOGRAM**

*A series of radiographs taken in rapid succession after a radio-opaque dye is injected into the coronary arteries. see Angiography.*

**ANGIOGRAPHY**

*An examination using a radio-opaque substance and X-rays to show the insides of the blood vessels.*

**ANGIOPLASTY**

*Form of surgery to repair, dilate or re-shape a damaged or blocked blood vessel.*

**ANGIOSCOPY**

*Examination in which a fibre optic tube is introduced into the blood vessels to give pictures of the inside on a television screen.*

**ANTICOAGULANT**

*Drug that prevents or stops the formation and/or extension of blood clots.*

**ANTIOXIDANT**

*Molecules that prevent the oxidation of bad cholesterol (LDL), thus reducing its harmful effects, as well as having many other functions.*

**AORTA**

*The main artery leaving the heart. It starts in the left ventricle and distributes oxygenated blood throughout the body. Other arteries in the body, including the coronary arteries, stem from the aorta.*

**ASPIRIN**

*Molecule (acetyl salicylic acid) with a pain-relieving and anti-inflammatory action; prevents platelets collecting together and for this reason is frequently used in the treatment of cardiovascular disease.*

**ATHEROMA**

*Fatty, fibrous and sometimes calcified deposits on the inner surface of artery walls. The thickness of these plaques increases with age.*

**ATHEROSCLEROSIS**

*Degenerative disease of the artery caused by the formation of atheroma plaques (fatty, fibrous and sometimes calcified deposits) on the artery wall. Atherosclerosis often leads to narrowing (stenosis), hardening and premature ageing of the arteries.*

**ATRIA (atrium in singular)**

*Heart cavities that receive blood before sending it through to the ventricles.*

**BACTERIA**

*The most widespread form of life on earth, and yet one of the most simple. Bacteria are single-cell organisms. Some are beneficial, others are pathogenic (they create diseases). Some bacteria may have a role in the cause of heart disease.*

**BETA-BLOCKERS**

*Drugs that counteract the effects of the hormones adrenaline and noradrenaline by attaching themselves to the body's receptors. They have anti-arrhythmic (irregularity of the heartbeat), anti-anginal and anti-hypertensive effects on the cardiovascular system.*

**BLOOD CELLS**

*There are three types, each with its own function. Red cells supply the body with oxygen; white cells protect against infection; and platelets help prevent heavy bleeding by forming blood clots.*

**BLOOD CLOT**

*Semi-solid mass made up of platelets and fibrin (which trap red and white cells), formed when blood coagulates. Clots prevent haemorrhaging when blood vessels are ruptured. They may form spontaneously (a thrombosis) inside the vessels and have serious consequences, causing phlebitis (inflammation of veins) or an embolism.*

**BLOOD PRESSURE**

*Pressure exerted on the blood vessels when the heart contracts and relaxes.*

**BLOOD PRESSURE, HIGH**

*Abnormal, permanent or paroxysmal (sudden) rise in blood pressure at rest. High blood pressure is defined by figures of 140/90 mm Hg or higher, but some experts believe we should be treating patients for high blood pressure when the reading is as low as 140/80.*

## C

**CARDIOMYOPATHY**

*From cardio (heart), myo (muscle) and pathy (disease). A generic term to describe any heart muscle disease.*

**CARDIOMYOPLASTY**

*Operation invented in France, consisting of placing part of a muscle from the back around the heart and contracting it electrically.*

**CATHETER**

Small plastic tube a few millimetres in diameter that can be pushed through the blood vessels.

**CHOLESTEROL**

Lipid or fat molecule, mostly synthesised by the liver and essential to the body. A high cholesterol level may lead to atherosclerosis and constitutes a cardiovascular risk.

**CORONARY ARTERIES**

Arteries arranged in a ring – hence their name – around the heart to ensure that it is well supplied with blood.

**DEFIBRILLATOR**

Machine that delivers an electric shock to the heart via two electrodes applied to the chest, with the aim of restoring the heart's normal rhythm.

**DIABETES**

When blood sugar level (or glycaemia) is too high. Diabetes is defined by a sugar level higher than 7.0 mmol/litre when fasting or 11.1 mmol/litre when not fasting on at least two occasions.

**DIASTOLE**

Period when the heart muscle is relaxed and the ventricles fill up with blood.

**DOPPLER**

An ultrasound examination used to measure the direction and velocity of blood flow through the heart or coronary arteries.

**ELECTROCARDIOGRAM**

Painless examination to analyse the heart's electrical activity. In most cases, it can reveal rhythm disorders, excess heart growth (hypertrophy), pericarditis, angina pectoris and infarction.

**EMBOLUS**

A mass (often a blood clot or piece of atheroma) which circulates in the blood and lodges in a different site from where it was produced.

**EMBOLISM**

Sudden obstruction of a vessel by a circulating embolus. After a heart attack, a clot may form inside the heart and then migrate through the circulatory system.

**ENDORPHIN**

Natural substance similar to morphine, synthesised in a variety of circumstances by some of the cells of the central nervous system. When in pain, some people synthesise more endorphin than others, which helps to explain why we all have different pain thresholds. Sporting activity and happiness seem to increase the synthesis of this protein.

**ENDOSCOPY**

Visual exploration of a body cavity, using an optic tube fitted with a lighting system, known as an endoscope or fibroscope.

**EXERTION TEST**

Examines the heart's electrical activity and how it functions during exertion. The exertion test helps diagnose coronary insufficiency.

**FATTY ACIDS
(or organic acids)**

These are the main constituents of lipids. There are more than 40 different fatty acids, differentiated according to how saturated or unsaturated they are. Saturated fatty acids can help cause atherosclerosis.

**FIBRILLATION, VENTRICULAR**

Very serious heart rhythm disorder leading to death; however, it can be immediately and effectively reversed by an electric shock to the heart (defibrillation), re-establishing normal heart rhythm.

**FIBRINOGEN**

An increased level of this protein constitutes a cardiovascular risk. This is manufactured in the liver and converted to harmful fibrin in damaged blood vessels.

**GLUCOSE**

Sugar or carbohydrate that is the greatest source of energy for the body's cells.

**GRAFT, VEIN**

Used during a heart bypass operation. The vein graft is taken from another vein in the patient himself (autograft).

**HDL**

HDL is High Density Lipoprotein, which is made of cholesterol and protein. Some blood cholesterol is transported as HDL, and some as LDL. HDL is known as good cholesterol, because it seems to protect against arterial disease. HDL cholesterol levels are as important as the total cholesterol level in estimating vascular risks.

**HEART**

Hollow muscular organ whose contractions ensure blood circulation throughout the body.

**HEART BYPASS**

Operation on the coronary arteries using a grafted vein or artery to bypass a blockage and thereby restore the blood supply to the heart.

# Glossary

## HEART ENZYMES

*Proteins liberated following the death or necrosis of heart cells during a heart attack.*

## HEPARIN

*Anticoagulant which may be injected into the veins or beneath the skin during the acute phase of a heart attack. It is also prescribed for the treatment and prevention of vein thrombosis and pulmonary embolism.*

## HOLTER MONITOR

*Examination that records the heart's electrical activity continuously for 24 hours (also known as 24-hour ambulatory ECG). Heart rhythm disorders during daily life can thus be discovered.*

## HOMOCYSTEINE

*An amino acid in the body; an increase in its level is considered to be a vascular risk factor.*

## IMAGING, MAGNETIC RESONANCE (MRI)

*Radiological technique providing very precise pictures of the body, using the magnetic vibrations of particles. These vibrations are picked up by a computer and turned into images.*

## INFARCTION

*Necrosis (death) in part of an organ, caused by a sudden failure of blood supply to that organ. A brain infarction leads to stroke; myocardial infarction (caused by coronary thrombosis) leads to necrosis in part of the heart; mesenteric infarction leads to necrosis in the intestine.*

## INSUFFICIENCY, CARDIAC

*Inability of the heart to carry out its work of pumping and propelling blood. This may affect the right side of the heart, the left side, or both.*

## INSUFFICIENCY, CORONARY

*Inability of the coronary arteries to supply enough oxygenated blood to the heart.*

## INSUFFICIENCY, MITRAL

*Fault in the closure of the mitral valve, causing blood to flow back from the left ventricle to the left atrium when the heart contracts.*

## ISCHAEMIA

*An inadequate flow of blood to part of an organ or area of tissue.*

## LDL

*Some cholesterol is transported as LDL (Low Density Lipoproteins). LDL may remain attached to the vascular walls. This bad cholesterol is a cardiovascular risk factor.*

## LIPID

*Fatty substance. Blood lipids include fatty acids, cholesterol, triglycerides and phospolipids.*

## LIPOPROTEIN (A)

*A protein and fat combination in the blood. This protein may represent a cardiovascular risk factor if its level in the blood increases.*

## LIPOPROTEIN

*Substance formed from a combination of proteins and lipids; ensures the transport of lipids in the blood.*

## MYOCARDIAL INFARCTION

*The medical name for a heart attack.*

## MYOCARDIUM

*Heart muscle. From myo (muscle), cardio (heart).*

## NECROSIS

*Death of a cell or organic tissue.*

## OESTROGEN

*Female sex hormone, secreted by the ovaries, that plays a role in ovulation and also protects the vascular walls against atherosclerosis.*

## PACEMAKER

*Mechanical heart stimulator that delivers electrical impulses to the myocardium, making it contract as soon as heart rate drops below a predetermined level.*

## PERICARDIUM

*Fibrous envelope surrounding the heart.*

## PERICARDITIS

*Inflammation of the pericardium, usually causing chest pain and moderate fever. May occur after a heart bypass operation. It can be treated with anti-inflammatories.*

## PLATELETS

*Blood cells that form clots to help the blood coagulate.*

## PRINZMETAL'S ANGOR

*Type of angina pectoris linked to a spasm in the coronary arteries. Occurs suddenly, often at night or at rest.*

## PULSE

*Rhythmic beating (pulsations) of the arteries as blood is pumped through them with every heart contraction. Heart rate can be measured by taking the pulse.*

**RESTENOSIS**

Formation of a new obstruction in a coronary artery despite angioplasty or a bypass.

**SCANNER**

Medical imaging machine using X-rays and linked to a computer. Gives precise pictures of the human body in fine cross-sections.

**SCINTIGRAPHY**

Medical imagery in which a radioactive dye, which has a strong affinity with a particular organ or tissue, is introduced into the body. Its uptake is recorded by a special camera.

**SEPTUM**

Part of the heart that divides the heart into right and left heart. It may be the site of an infarction.

**STENOSIS**

A dangerous narrowing of the diameter of a blood vessel or orifice.

**STENOSIS, AORTIC**

A harmful narrowing of the aortic valve opening.

**STENT (coronary)**

Wire mesh tube placed, during angioplasty, at the site of a coronary artery stenosis to keep the vessel.

**STROKE**

Usual name for a cerebral vascular accident, brain infarction or cerebral haemorrhage, which may lead to paralysis (hemiplegia).

**SYNTHESISE**

To make within the body.

**SYSTOLE**

Phase during which the heart contracts, propelling blood towards the lungs, the aorta and the rest of the body.

**TACHYCARDIA**

Acceleration of heart rate beyond 100 beats per minute.

**THROMBOLYSIS**

From the Greek thrombos (clot) and lyse (destruction). Destruction of a clot using drugs called thrombolytics.

**THROMBOLYTICS**

Very powerful anticoagulant drugs, used to destroy intravascular blood clots rapidly.

**THROMBOSIS**

Formation of a blood clot (called a thrombus) in an artery or vein.

**TRANSPLANT, HEART**

Transplanting the heart of a deceased donor into a patient.

**TRIGLYCERIDE**

One of the lipids circulating in the blood. The level may be increased by many things, such as hereditary factors, alcoholism, diabetes or the taking of contraceptives.

**TRINITROGLYCERIN**

Chemical substance derived from nitrous acid. A powerful vasodilator, which opens up blood vessels, used to treat angina pectoris.

**ULTRASOUND, HEART**

Anatomical and functional examination of the heart, using ultrasound waves. These are reflected by the heart muscle and turned into images.

**ULTRASOUND, TRANS-OESOPHAGAL (TOU)**

Heart ultrasound using an ultrasound probe inserted down the oesophagus, and just behind the heart. This enables doctors to see any blood clots inside the heart and can also show up an aneurism on the aorta.

**VALVES**

The heart valves are four segmented membranes channelling blood through the heart, ensuring that it only flows in one direction.

**VASODILATING DRUGS**

Drugs that increase the diameter of blood vessels.

**VENAE CAVAE**

The two largest veins in the body, the superior vena cava and the inferior vena cava join to the right atrium, returning venous blood to the heart.

**VENTRICLES**

Heart cavities that propel blood into the lungs (role of the right ventricle) and into the aorta (role of the left ventricle).

**VITAMINS**

Organic substances needed for the growth and healthy functioning of the body. Some are synthesised in the body, others have to be supplied by our food. Some may play an important role in the prevention of atherosclerosis: vitamins, C, E, B1, B₆ and folic acid.

**XENOGRAFTING**

Grafting animal tissue into humans.

# Contents

# Fact ⫸ 2–12
Fun facts and quick quotes

# Discover ⫸ 13–34

# Look ⫸ 35–52
Colourful images get to the heart of the matter

# In practice ⫸ 53–92

# Find out ⟫ 93–125

# Credits

**p8 and 45**, *Le Sacré Coeur de Marie* Central European lithograph, c.1900, private collection, photo Jean-Louis Charmet. **p14**, The heart and the organs in the chest, lithograph by Haincelin in *Manual of descriptive anatomy* by J. Cloquet, Paris 1825, photo Jean-Louis Charmet. **p16** Weighing the heart, detail from a page of *The Book of the Dead* , an Egyptian papyrus, Paris, Louvre, The Bridgeman Art Library, photo Peter Willi. **p19** , Human sacrifice in an Aztec temple, 16th century manuscript, Florence: Medici Library, The Bridgeman Art Library. **p20** Hippocrates, engraving, Paris, BNF, © Harlingue/Viollet. **p22** Anatomical drawing of the heart and blood vessels, Leonardo da Vinci, private collection, The Bridgeman Art Library. **p24** William Harvey, Paris: BNF © Roger/Viollet. **p27** Sphygmographs in *La Vie normale et la santé* by Dr Rengade, Paris, 1881, photo Jean-Louis Charmet. **p29** *The cardiologist, H. Vaquez, and his assistant* , painting by Edouard Vuillard circa 1917, Paris: Musée de l'Assistance Publique, photo Jean-Louis Charmet. **p30**, Coronarography, operational radiography dept. under Pr. Didier Revel, Hôpital Cardiologique de Lyon, © P. Alix/Phanie. **p33**, Defibrillator implant, © J-P Joubert/Phanie. **pp36–37**, © Sitko/Explorer. **p38** © P. Le Floch/Explorer. **p39** © B. Annebique/Sygma. **p40**, © Thouvenin/Explorer. **pp42–43**, Heart-shaped world map by Orontius, 1536, Paris: BNF, AKG photo. **p46**, © R. Chapple/Misc/General. **p47**, Photo Terry Jones, The Bridgeman Art Library. **p48**, ©Roland and Sabina Michaud. **p49**, © Paul M. Tatopoulos/Explorer. **p51**, © G. Rancinan/Sygma. **p52**, © Abbas/Magnum. **pp54–57**, 60–62, 64–72, 74, 77–92, Infographs: Laurent Rullier. **p58**, © *Science et Vie* . **p63**, Atheroma seen by ultrasound-Doppler, © BSIP CMSP. **p63**, Atheroma plaque on the wall of the carotid artery, © GJLP CNRI. **p69**, Aneurism on the abdominal aorta, © Airelle/Joubert – Phanie. **p73**, Heart echodoppler, © J-P Joubert/Phanie. **p95**, © Stills. **pp96–113** and **116–119**, Illustrations:Philippe Andrieux. **pp114–115**, illustration: Laurent Blachier.

# Acknowledgements

The authors would like to thank Doctor Yves Esanu for his invaluable advice and Jacqueline Vallon for her collaboration.

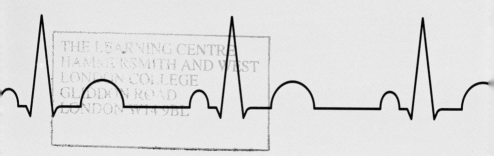